14

OPHTHALMIC TECHNICAL SKILLS SERIES

Ophthalmic Photography

Revised Edition

J. Michael Coppinger, MA, CRA
Mark Maio
Kirby Miller, CRA

SLACK Incorporated, 6900 Grove Road, Thorofare, New Jersey 08086

SLACK International Book Distributors

In Canada:
McGraw-Hill Ryerson Limited
330 Progress Avenue
Scarborough, Ontario
M1P 2Z5

In Australia and New Zealand:
MacLennan & Petty Pty Limited
P.O. Box 425
Artarmon, N.S.W. 2064
Australia

In Japan:
Igaku-Shoin, Ltd.
Tokyo International P.O. Box 5063
1-28-36 Hongo, Bunkyo-Ku
Tokyo 113
Japan

In Asia and India:
PG Publishing Pte Limited.
36 West Coast Road, #02-02
Singapore 0512

Foreign Translation Agent

John Scott & Company
International Publishers' Agency
417-A Pickering Road
Phoenixville, PA 19460
Fax: 215-988-0185

Managing Editor: Lynn C. Borders
Designer: Susan Hermansen
Production Manager: David Murphy
Publisher: Harry C. Benson

Printed in the United States of America

Library of Congress Catalog Card Number: 90-053188

ISBN: 1-55642-170-2
Ophthalmic Technical Skills Series, Volume I ISBN: 1-55642-044-7

Published by: SLACK Incorporated
6900 Grove Road
Thorofare, NJ 08086

Last digit is print number: 10 9 8 7 6 5 4 3 2 1

About This Series

The field of Ophthalmic Medical Assisting has been developing since the early 1960s. Initially assistants were hired as scribes; but as new technology was introduced, more technical tasks were delegated to office personnel in order to mobilize the physician for a more high-tech examination and treatment role. Each year a greater number of advanced technologies filter down to technical personnel, who need to be competently trained. In order to meet this demand for education, various formal educational programs for the Ophthalmic Medical Assistant have been developed; and to date ten programs in the United States are accredited by the American Medical Association. Various organizations participating in the Joint Commission on Allied Health Personnel in Ophthalmology have collaborated to define the three technical levels (assistant, technician, technologist) and continued to update the criteria for certification of each level.

With the goals of quality care for the patient and professional enjoyment for the ophthalmic team, we will approach the turn of the twenty-first century more successfully with education. All members of the ophthalmic team constantly need to sharpen their clinical expertise, acumen, and awareness in order to identify serious pathology outside the daily routine of the practice. This attention to detail enhances the quality of care we want for our patients and the professional confidence gained from a job well done. It requires a broad education, which includes a general understanding of anatomy, disease, diagnosis, and management, and a set of ready references to remind us of key concepts and methods. This series is designed to update and supplement your current knowledge. It is a reference guide to help the beginner as well as the experienced practitioner and those reviewing for their certification.

Candace P. Wolfe, MEd., COMT
Formerly, Director of
Ophthalmic Technology Program
Scheie Eye Institute
University of Pennsylvania

Susan C. Benes, MD
Department of Ophthalmology
Ohio State University

About This Series

To my wife

Luisa

who still loves me after this enormous effort

J. Michael

Contents

About The Authors

The three authors of this book are all practicing clinical ophthalmic photographers, all actively engaged in teaching their skills to others.

J. Michael Coppinger, the principal author, is an active professional ophthalmic photographer with fifteen years of experience in his specialized field. He directed the ophthalmic photography unit in the Department of Ophthalmology at Pacific Presbyterian Medical Center in San Francisco for nine years. He is currently owner-operator of JMC Eye Photo, a business expressly devoted to ophthalmic photographic training.

Mark Maio is assistant clinical professor in the Department of Ophthalmology at the State University of New York at Buffalo. Mr. Maio was previously director of Ophthalmic Photography at Emory Eye Center in Atlanta for seven years.

Kirby Miller is the ophthalmic photographer at the University of Mississippi Medical Center at Jackson, Mississippi. He was previously a research assistant in the Department of Ophthalmology for nine years at Tulane Medical School in New Orleans.

All three gentlemen are members of the Ophthalmic Photographers Society. They teach at both OPS and JCAHPO annual meetings. All three conduct training courses throughout the United States as faculty members of JMC Eye Photo. All three have been guest faculty at numerous other opthalmology and ophthalmic photography courses throughout the United States.

The authors' desire to teach photography created this book. The forty-five collective years of experience in the field of ophthalmic photography mothered it. The patience of three wonderful wives, Luisa Coppinger, Catherine Maio, and Donna Miller, nourished it. The authors trust the readers will benefit from it.

Foreword

Ophthalmic photography began as an adjunct to the field of ophthalmology when Dr. Noyce took the first photographs of the retina of a rabbit in 1862. Nearly a century later, a series of ingenious experiments using fluorescein dye led to the development of a new diagnostic technique in ophthalmology: fluorescein angiography. Along the way have been innumerable individuals who have helped pave the way to make ophthalmic photography the field it is today. John Michael Coppinger, in my mind, exemplifies the best of these individuals.

With the advent of ophthalmic photography as a profession, the ophthalmic photographer has increasingly assumed the role of both photographer and educator. Mr. Coppinger has been at the forefront of ophthalmic photography education. He has served as the Chief of Ophthalmic Photography at Pacific Presbyterian Medical Center in San Francisco for many years. He has also run widely acclaimed instruction courses for photographers and physicians throughout the country.

I would be remiss, however, if I were to limit my comments about Mr. Coppinger to the field of ophthalmic photography alone. His training in photography at the John Vickers School of Photography in London attests to his interest in the field of photography as a whole. It seems fitting to me that one of the great ophthalmic photographers of our time applies his expertise in photography to, not just the eyes, but to all that is around us. It is with the help of such individuals that we all get to see a world in a new light.

Everett Ai, M.D.
Director, Retina Service
Pacific Presbyterian Medical
Center, San Francisco, California

Preface

We have written this book to provide a resource.

The book you are about to read was written to introduce you to the technical aspects of ophthalmic photography. This book is primarily a how to book with explanation.

We've begun with the basic principles of photography, and then applied these principles to each type of ophthalmic photography used in clinical practice today.

No book, of course, can offer the hands-on experience you'll need to master these techniques. As you follow the instructions and advice outlined, you'll make errors which drive home many points made here. Hopefully the authors' experience will help minimize these pitfalls.

As teachers and authors, we welcome suggestions for inclusion in the second edition of this volume. Please write with any comments or questions.

Stay in focus,

J. Michael Coppinger, Mark Maio, Kirby Miller
Shaftsbury, Vermont October, 1987

CHAPTER 1

Photographic Principles

by J. Michael Coppinger

Ophthalmic photography is a branch of the more general craft of photography. This subspecialty concentrates on the recording of images to document various pathological conditions of the human eye. As we will see in the chapters that follow, there are many special types of ophthalmic photography, each used to record a different part of the human eye.

Before we explore each of these photographic techniques, we will define some general photographic terms and explain the principles involved in making a picture. This background is essential to understand the descriptions of ophthalmic photographic techniques.

Photography, from the Greek "photos" and "graphos," means light writing. Four basic components are necessary to record and store a permanent image: light, camera, film, and development.

Light

Light is electromagnetic radiation moving through space that can evoke a human visual response. Photons of energy move outward from a light source in all directions. As these photons move they oscillate back and forth in a wave pattern. The measure from peak A to peak A_1 of the wave oscillation is the wavelength of a particular color of light radiation (Figure 1.1).

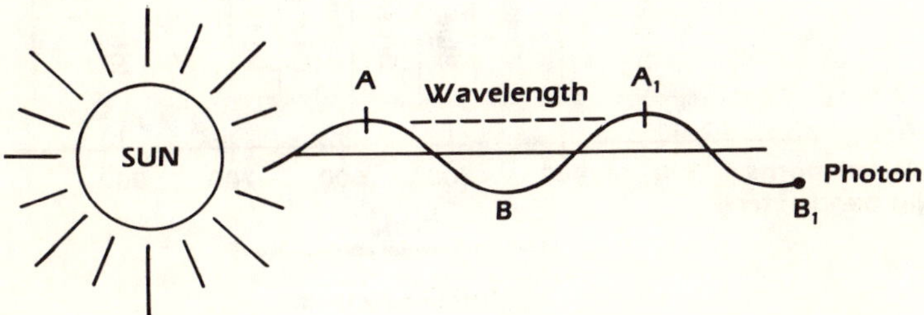

Figure 1.1 The wavelength of a light ray is the measure of oscillation of a light photon from peak (A) to peak (A^1) as it proceeds away from the energy source—here, the sun.

The light reflected by a unit area of any surface in a particular direction is called luminance. Luminance is measured in candles/square foot with photoelectric meters to compute correct photographic exposures. Other than loss by reflection or absorption, luminance is unchanged by an optical system. Luminance is measurable light.

All energy sources, from atomic radiation to television signals, follow this same general pattern of wave oscillation. Wavelengths are measured in meters or parts of meters. Light is measured in billionths of a meter, or **nanometers.** The term "visible light" is redundant. Light is radiant energy we can see with our eyes. Light has a wavelength range from 400 nanometers to 700 nanometers. This range is called the **visible spectrum.** Conventional colors are associated with specific wavelengths ranging from blue (400–490 N) to green (490–560 N) to yellow (560–610 N) to red (640–700 N) (Figure 1.2).

Wavelengths shorter than 400 N are of a higher energy. This energy is called **ultraviolet.** Wavelengths longer than 700 N are called **infrared.** While the eye cannot see these radiations, we can use camera and film to record them, and often refer to them as ultraviolet and infrared "light."

Natural Light

The most common photographic light we encounter is daylight, the light of the sun and sky. Daylight contains all the wavelengths of the spectrum, that is, all colors. The color of an object we perceive is the wavelength of light reflected from that object. Thus a red rose is reflecting red wavelengths to our eyes. Black objects absorb all wavelengths of light, while white objects reflect all wavelengths.

Daylight can be recreated by using a light source that emanates or emits the entire spectrum of light. There are two light sources commonly used to re-create daylight. One is the photo flash bulb—a sealed glass housing in which a metal filament explodes in an oxygen-filled glass bulb emitting a high-intensity light radiation. A second type is the electronic flash unit, in which an instantaneous electric discharge between two electrodes is produced through an atmosphere of inert gas, usually xenon. Most ophthalmic units use some type of electronic flash unit or tube.

Flash bulbs can be used only once, while electronic flashes use AC current or batteries and will continue to operate as

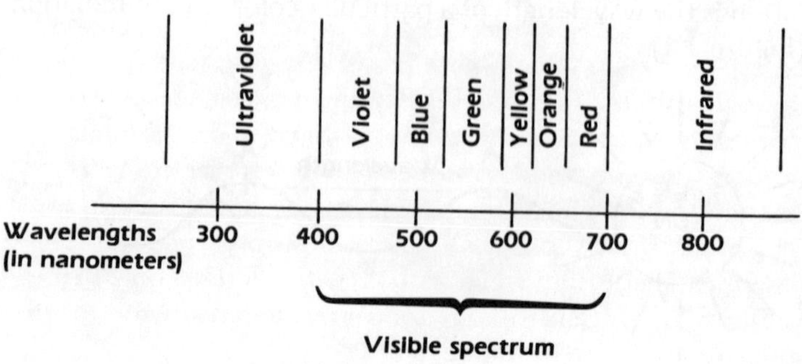

Figure 1.2 The spectrum of light represented in nanometers (billionths of a meter).

long as an energy source is available to fire them. Such artificial devices for creating daylight allow accurate, full-spectrum color rendition in artificial light.

Panchromatic—meaning all colors—films are manufactured to be light sensitive to the entire visible spectrum. Such films and photographic papers must be loaded for development in total darkness. Orthochromatic films can be developed in red light, as these films are only sensitive to blue and green light. Black-and-white photographic papers are made sensitive to either yellow or red light, but not both.

Artificial Light

Artificial light is light that is not produced by the sun. There are three common artificial light sources used in photography. The first is the electronic flash unit. The second is the photo flood or conventional tungsten light bulb. This source of light contains primarily red wavelengths, with little green or blue light (Figure 1.3). The human eye and brain adjust for this abnormal color balance, seeing such an illuminated scene as "normally" colored. Film sees and records this disparity in color saturation. Most ophthalmic instruments use tungsten light sources for illumination viewing. Quartz halogen lamps are tungsten lamps.

The third type of artifical light source is the fluorescent light bulb. This phosphorous-lined glass tube containing mercury vapor has an electric charge constantly moving through it to excite and emit light radiation. Fluorescent light is irregular in spectral composition, containing four peaks of red, green, and blue radiation, which correspond to the mercury radiation spectral emission, as well as a weaker continous spectrum radiation from the phosphor lining of the tube. Fluorescent light is not frequently used in ophthalmic photography.

All types of artificial light can be transmitted through fiber optic tubes, in which light is conducted through a bundle of threadlike pieces of glass or plastic by means of total internal reflection, so that an image formed at one end will emerge from the other end even though the bundle is curved. The spectrum of light passed through a fiber optic tube can be controlled by the user. Later we will see that fiber optics play a role in a special type of retinal photography.

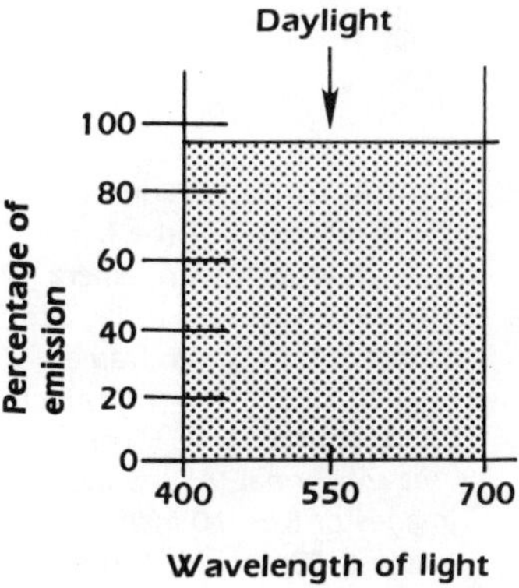

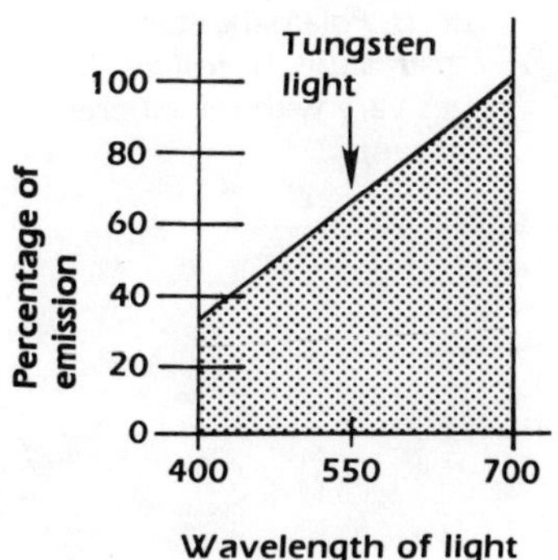

Figure 1.3 The relative concentration of spectral emission of daylight (top) and a conventional tungsten light bulb (bottom).

The Camera

Light falling on the surface of the subject we choose to photograph is the same light we wish to record as a permanent image, i.e., a picture. To do this, we need a mechanical device—a camera—containing a light-sensitive material—film. Our own eyes are the model for this mechanical device we will create to trap light and then process it to make an image or picture. Observe the details as we first describe camera and film and then relate each part or function to the human eye.

Camera (from the Latin) means a room. A photographic camera is a light-tight room (or box) with a lens or hole in one wall and a light-sensitive material positioned on the inside opposite wall. The human eye is also a room that contains a

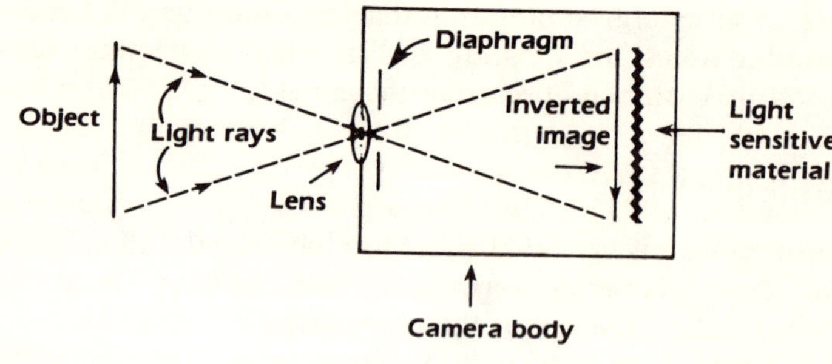

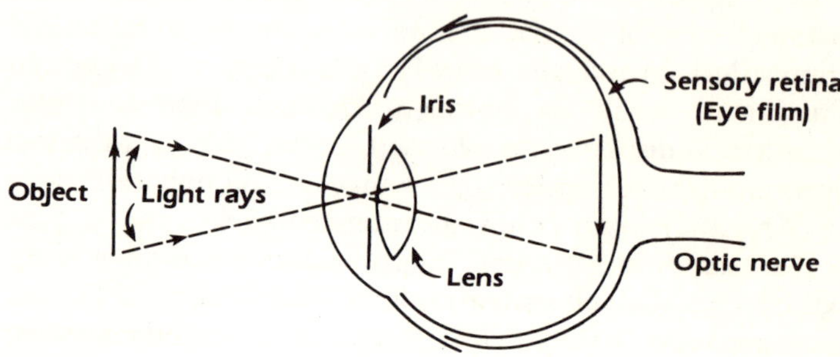

Figure 1.4 A simple box camera (top). The eye as a camera (bottom).

Camera format designates the dimensions of the film used in a particular camera. Standard film sizes today are 35mm (24 × 36mm framed image), 120 (2 1/4 × 2 1/4 inch images), and "4 × 5" or "view" format (4 × 5 inch images or 8 × 10 inch images). 35mm and 120 formats use roll film. View format uses individual film sheets. Polaroid instant cameras use sheet films (film sizes vary with the different systems).

light-sensitive material—the sensory retina—with its nerves, rods, and cones (Figure 1.4). In front of the lens in the eye is a diaphragm—the iris—acting as a hole that opens wide enough to allow light rays to pass through and strike the retinal "film," thus fixing the image of the object or scene in focus. In a camera, a light energy image is stored or captured by the photographic film as a latent (invisible) image of electrically charged photons. After exposure—the act of letting light reach the film—is completed, the photographic film is removed from the camera and chemically developed to render the latent image visible. The human eye develops the image by passing a chemical signal through the optic nerve to the brain for processing (or development). We call this development "sight."

Photographic cameras can contain numerous mechanical features, such as shutters, focusing mechanisms, interchangeable lenses, film backs, viewfinders, and built-in light meters to compute exposure. The human brain provides some of these functions for the eyes. Keep the human eye in mind as we anatomize the photographic camera.

The Simplest Camera Does Not Even Need a Lens

In 1039 an Arabian scholar, Alhazen, demonstrated that light from one room would pass through a hole in a wall into an adjoining room to produce an inverted image of the lighted room on a hand-held piece of white paper in the light ray's path. This "pinhole" camera was refined in the 1500s in box form and used by artists for sketching paintings. This so-called "camera obscura" was refined by the addition of a lens by Gardano in 1550. The subsequent refinement of optics in the 1500s and the development of chemistry (1600–1800), and physics (Newton) provided the building blocks for direct formation and recording of images as we know it today.

In ophthalmic photography, the common camera format (size of film) used is 35mm; this produces an image in the camera 24mm × 36mm on the film. Vertical and horizontal dimensions are determined by the positioning of the camera. The term 35mm refers to the width across the roll of film. Sprockets on either side of the roll allow easy transport of film through the camera.

There are two types of conventional 35mm cameras. One is the **rangefinder** camera. Rangefinder cameras are body-box cameras with an optical rangefinder mounted on top and interconnected to the focusing mechanism. The photographer looks through the rangefinder port at the subject. By adjusting the focus mechanism a small part of the viewed image (produced by additional optics, either mirrors or prisms) moves relative to the larger image. Exact focus is achieved when the two images overlap. Rangefinders focus by scale, and can be used to measure camera-to-subject distance without moving.

Rangefinder cameras are poorly suited to close up (macro) photography. Because the viewport is separate from the camera lens the actual image photographed does not coincide with the one seen on the viewfinder. This effect is called **parallax.** Rangefinder cameras also show less in the viewfinder than is recorded on the film. The rangefinder, for these reasons, is not widely used in ophthalmic photography.

The more widely used type of 35mm camera is the **single lens reflex** (SLR) camera, so called because the lens used to make the photograph is also used, by the interposition of a moving mirror, to form an image on a ground glass screen on top of the camera to focus this same image. "Reflex" could be more accurately be stated as reflecting. The light from the lens reflects off the mirror onto a ground glass plate. A three-way penta-prism placed over the ground glass reflects the light to the photographer's eye for composition and focus. When the shutter is triggered to make a photograph, the mirror swings out of the light path to the film. When exposure is complete, the mirror returns to its original position.

Use of the same lens to focus and make photos eliminates the problem of parallax. Close-up photography is easily accomplished using the SLR camera. Exact framing in the viewfinder allows full use of the film frame.

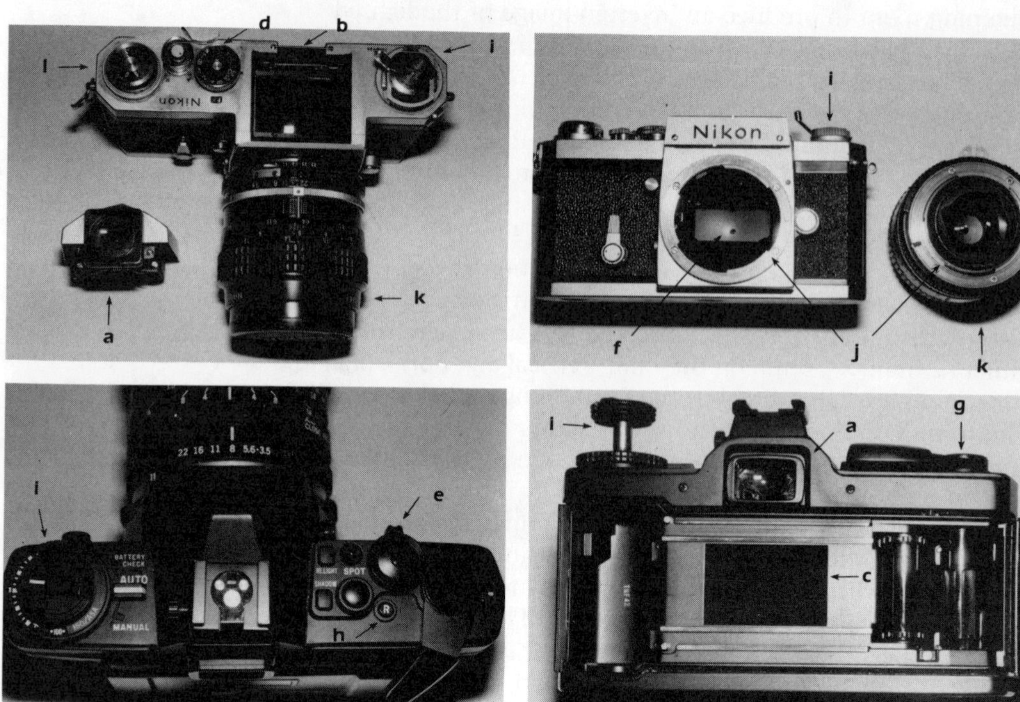

Figure 1.5 Main components of a 35 mm camera: (a) viewfinder (b) viewing screen (c) shutter (d) shutter speed (e) shutter release (f) eyepiece mirror (g) film advance (h) rewind button (i) rewind knob (j) lens mount (k) lens (l) frame counter.

The single lens reflex camera is the one conventionally used in ophthalmic photography so we shall delineate its main features in greater detail.

SLR cameras contain certain basic components subdivided into camera body and camera lenses.

The **camera body** contains eleven common features. As most ophthalmic cameras use conventional 35 millimeter (mm) bodies and film, delineation in some detail of these eleven features is necessary (Figure 1.5).

A common feature of the modern 35mm camera is the light meter, also called the exposure meter. This meter is a photoelectric instrument used to measure luminance for correct exposure of the film. Fully automated cameras not only measure, but also calculate mathematically correct exposure and display both time and aperture to be used on a scale with the camera viewfinder.

The Viewfinder

The viewfinder displays how much of the subject will be included in the photograph. The photographer looks through the viewfinder to see the subject. Viewfinders are usually built into the camera optics but they may be separate optical systems. On certain fundus cameras there is a separate eyepiece viewfinder.

The Viewing Screen

The viewing screen is a piece of ground glass in the viewfinder of the camera body. The image to be photographed is displayed on this screen, and proper focus is created by adjusting a focus mechanism until the image on the screen is sharp. These viewing screens can often be removed from the standard camera body and exchanged for a screen with a different type of focusing aid. For conventional 35mm camera lens combination systems, refer to your camera manual for more information on the viewfinder.

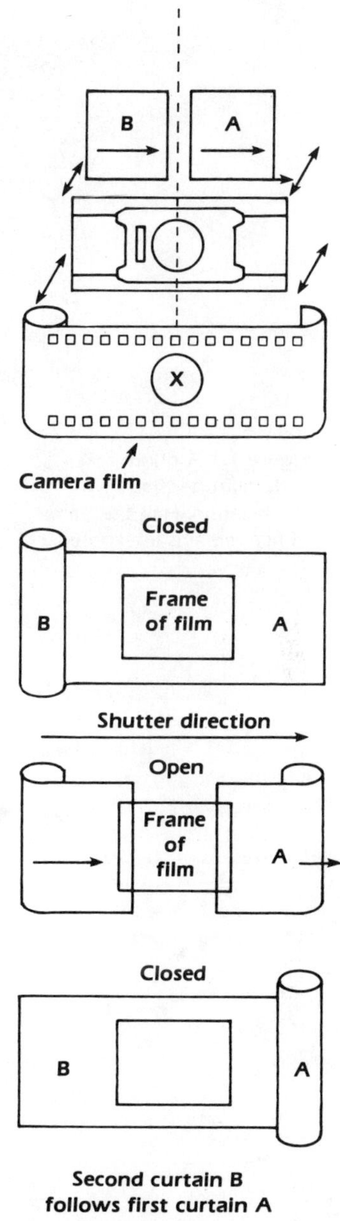

Figure 1.6 The action of a focal plane shutter.

The Shutter

The shutter is a mechanical device for controlling the duration the film in the camera is exposed to light. There are two common types of shutters, the leaf diaphragm shutter and the focal plane shutter. The leaf shutter has a set of overlapping metal blades that open together toward the outer circumference of the shutter leaving a central hole for light to pass to the film. Such shutters are independent camera parts that can be positioned either in front of or behind the lens of the camera. Older camera systems, especially large format (4″ × 5″) view cameras employ this type of shutter.

The more commonly used shutter in 35mm photography is the focal plane shutter (Figure 1.6). This shutter consists of two opaque screens (blinds) with a slit between them that move from one side to the other immediately in front of the focal plane of the lens. (The focal plane is the hypothetical flat surface that represents the focus of an infinitely distant flat object surface perpendicular to the lens axis, i.e., the image plane where the film is positioned in the camera body.) This shutter may move either up, down, or across in front of the focal plane. The time of an exposure is determined by the distance between the blinds, and the speed at which they cross the rollers, the tracks on which the blinds move. The slit exposes sequentially the frame or unit of exposed film as it travels across. The lag between the first and second slide is the duration of exposure.

Such shutters have speed ranges from 1 second to $^1/_{2000}$ of a second. These speeds are displayed on the shutter speed dial. Focal plane shutters often include a T or B setting which allows opening the blinds to expose all the film at once and holding the shutter open as long as the shutter release is held open.

A second feature of such shutters is the flash synchronization setting. This is the shortest time setting of the shutter that will allow full frame exposure when using electronic flash. This time setting is usually $^1/_{60}$ or $^1/_{125}$ of a second. It is marked with an X on the shutter speed control, dial indicating the setting for flash synchronization. Using too fast a shutter speed produces images with only part of the image exposed, because the shutter opens and closes more quickly than the duration of the flash (Figure 1.7)

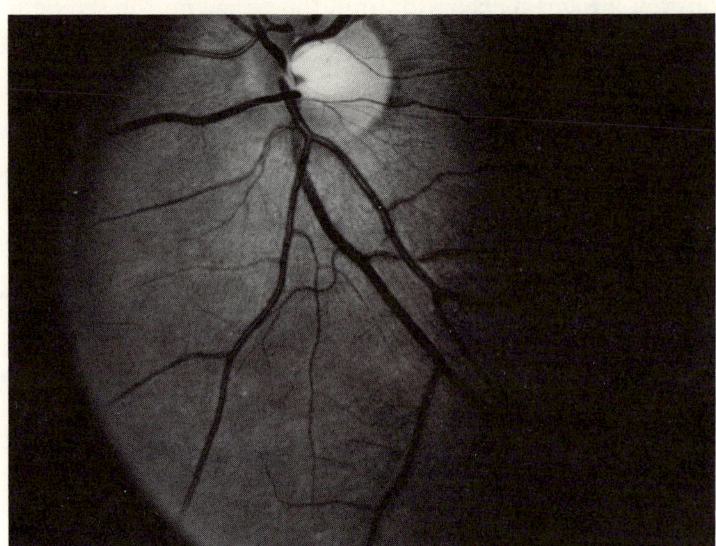

Figure 1.7 A photo taken with improper flash synchronization. Half the frame of film remains unexposed.

Shutter Speed Dial

The shutter speed dial sets the speed of shutter operation. Speed ranges vary from camera to camera but all follow a conventional geometric progression, that is, each speed is double or half the previous one. Shutter speeds progress from $1/_{1000}$ second to 1, 2, or 4 full seconds. In ophthalmic photography, electronic flash exposure is the rule in almost all applications, so shutter speed on a camera body should be set to the flash synchronization setting, (usually $1/_{60}$ of a second). Some ophthalmic camera bodies operate only at a shutter speed preset for electronic flash, and have no shutter speed dial. Always read the manual of the camera being used to get the exact setting for flash synchronization.

Shutter Release

Flash refers to flash bulbs, flash lamps and elecronic flash. Only electronic flash is conventionally used in ophthalmic photography. Flash duration is much shorter than shutter speed when synchronized mechanically so the full surge of light can be captured on film. Flash will synchronize at all speeds slower than flash setting (x).

The shutter release is the button that, when pressed, initiates the exposure of the film. Usually this release is located on the camera body. Cable releases can be attached to such buttons to allow remote triggering of the shutter. These releases are used during long exposures to avoid camera movement. Such remote releases can be locked to hold the shutter open for long time exposures. Remote releases are also useful in operating room photography to avoid field contamination by the photographer. Shutters on many ophthalmic photo camera systems are electronically wired to firing buttons located on the "joystick," the lever that controls movement of the camera base and support. Pressing the button located on this control mechanism triggers the flash exposure system of the camera.

Eyepiece Mirror

The eyepiece mirror is positioned in front of the shutter to divert the image forming light entering the camera lens through a series of prisms to the viewfinder to allow composition of an image. When the shutter is released to make an exposure, the mirror moves upward out of the light path to the film to allow the image to be recorded.

Film Transport Advance Mechanism

The film transport advance mechanism is used to manually advance the film through the camera after each exposure. When the shutter has been released, this lever is rotated to move the next frame of unexposed film into position for exposure. The film advance lever is geared to the film winding spool. Many ophthalmic cameras feature a motorized automatic film transport that advances the film in the camera one frame after each exposure. When one manually advances the film, one should rotate the lever counterclockwise until meeting resistance. The shutter release will again operate once the film has been fully advanced. This feature prevents double exposures in the camera.

Rewind Mechanism

The rewind mechanism has two parts. The button, usually on the camera bottom, releases the film advance transport mechanism's gears, and allows the film to be rewound into the film cassette after exposure. The other part is the rewind knob, which one rotates counterclockwise to draw the film back into its cassette. Many motorized 35mm cameras have a button on the motor drive unit that also must be correctly positioned to allow either film advance or rewind. Check the manual.

Frame Counter

The frame counter is an indicator, usually on the top or back of the camera body, which displays how many frames of film have been (additive counter) or remain to be (subtractive counter) exposed.

The Lens Mount

The lens mount is a device on the front of the camera body

that holds or attaches the lens to the camera body, or ophthalmic camera instrument.

Camera Back Door

The camera back door is a hinged door with its own release mechanism that opens to allow access to the inside of the camera body to load and unload film. Check the manual for specific operating instructions on each camera you use. Be sure that this door is tightly closed after you load film into a camera back to prevent light from leaking in and damaging the film moving through the camera as pictures are taken.

Check the instructions for the specific camera you are using. While many camera bodies feature additional useful devices, the devices outlined here are the critical features necessary on most camera bodies.

Camera Lenses

The second major component of a camera system is the **lens.**

Simply defined, a lens is an optical device, usually made of glass or plastic, for forming an image of an object by the refraction of light.

There are two types of photographic lenses—converging and diverging. (For more specifics on **refraction,** consult the Optics book in this series.)

Converging lenses bend parallel rays of light to bring them together to a point of focus located on the opposite side of the lens (Figure 1.8). Converging lenses are positive lenses.

Diverging lenses bend parallel rays of light away from one another on the opposite side of the lens so they appear to originate from a single point in front of the lens. Diverging lenses are negative lenses. Lenses are composed of single or compound elements or parts. A single lens is one composed of a single piece of glass (or other material). A compound lens

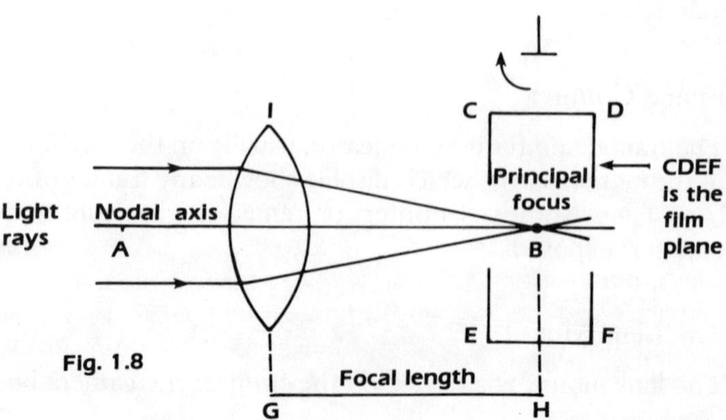

Figure 1.8 A converging lens with its two principal foci (A + B). CDEF represent the focal plane of the camera film—a real image.

is one with more than one optical element, the multiplc parts each working to correct the imperfections of another of its component parts. Complex lenses often combine converging and diverging lens elements.

The light ray that passes through the center of a lens is called the axis.

Most conventional cameras, as well as ophthalmic photographic instruments, use compound lenses. The optical properties of the material used to make the lens has a direct bearing on its resolution of detail. Lenses can be coated to aid in resolution. Ophthalmic instrument lens systems usually magnify the subject size on the film, consequently the optical quality of the lenses is very high (and expensive).

All lenses have the same basic optical relationships. A line drawn perpendicularly through the center of a lens about which all radii are symmetrical is called the lens axis or the nodal axis (Figure 1.8). When light rays from a great distance pass through a converging lens, they all bend inward to a common point on the nodal axis called the principal focus. With diverging lenses, light passing through the lens bends outward appearing to originate on the other side of the lens, again its principal focus. Converging lenses produce real points of real images that can be projected and focused on a screen. Diverging lenses, however, produce no real projectable images, so we differentiate diverging lens images as virtual images.

Light can pass through lenses in both directions, so it follows that for each direction light travels there is a principal focus for a specific lens, that is, all lenses have two principal foci. If we draw flat planes at right angles to the lens axis at the principal foci of the lens, we have principal focal planes for our lens (the position of the film in the camera). As a photographic convention, the front surface of a lens faces the subject, the back surface the film. If the lens is focused on an object at infinity, the subject's plane of focus is sharply imaged on the rear principal plane of focus, the film. By building a camera body so that the photographic film is placed in this plane, we can achieve sharply focused images with our camera. By racking the lens on an adjustable focusing ring, which we can mechanically move forward and backward, we can adjust the lens focus to subjects closer than infinity and refract the light striking our subject to sharp focus on the rear focal plane, that is, focus our image.

Lenses can be either flat surfaced, spheric or aspheric (nonspheric). Conventional camera lenses are usually spheric. However, in the fundus camera used for retinal photography we use aspheric lenses (see Chapter 5). An aspheric lens has one or more nonspherical surfaces, which can often produce optically superior images.

The lens of the human eye has a property unlike any optical lens—the ability to change shape with focus. This ability is called accomodation. As the human eye changes focus from a far point to a near point the lens changes from a flat, thin shape to a rounder, thicker one. As we age, the elasticity of our lenses diminishes, and additional lenses (glasses) become necessary to focus at near points. A camera lens changes focus by moving the lens forward and backward in relation to the position of the film.

The human eye contains an adjustable aperture, the iris. This aperture is automatically adjustable to light conditions, opening in darker areas, stopping down to pinhole size in bright areas. This involuntary neural changing of the iris' aperture can be adjusted pharmacologically with dilating drops. Maximum pupil aperture is mandatory for retinal photography. Dilation also paralyzes patient lens accommodation, fixing the optics of their lens in a relaxed, thin shape.

All lenses have specific focal lengths. The focal length of a lens is the measured distance (usually in mm) from the center point of the lens to the principal focal point on the lens axis (Figure 1.8). Light rays from infinity focused through the lens are most sharp at this distance. The focal length determines image size at a given lens-to-subject distance. Books on lenses and optics delineate in great detail formulas for creating and measuring focal lengths in lenses.

A 35mm camera with a normal lens has a focal length of 50mm; 35mm lenses of longer focal length (75mm to 400mm) are called telephoto lenses. These lenses are optically longer, and magnify the image size on the film and restrict the angle of view from edge-to-edge of the subject in the viewfinder. Shorter focal length lenses (24mm to 40mm) reduce magnification while expanding angle of view and are called wide angle lenses. With all ophthalmic camera lens systems, whether external, slit lamp, specular, or retinal camera, each change in magnification either up or down has an inverse effect on the angle of view of the subject. The higher the magnification (focal length) the narrower the angle of view.

The normal camera lens also needs a control, called the aperture, to allow a measured amount of light to pass through the lens. The size of the aperture (pupil) can be fixed or adjustable. Conventional camera lenses have leaf diaphragms attached to an *aperture* ring control that allows the user to open up or close down the aperture. The aperture ring operates geometrically (like the shutter speed dial) doubling or halving as we open or close it by measured amounts. These graduated adjustments are uniformly standardized and referred to as *f-numbers*. The largest aperture opening in the standard number sequence is f1, each subsequent number f 1.4, 2, 2.8, 4, 5.6, 8, 11, 16, 22, 32 being one half the area of the previous number, hence passing half as much light (Figure 1.9). A lens receives its f number from the largest diameter opening the aperture can achieve. Sometimes this number lies between two numbers on the standard scale, as with for example a 55mm focal length lens with a maximum aperture of f3.5. The larger the aperture f-number for a given focal length lens, the greater "speed" of the lens, that is, the more light passing through the lens. Shutter speed and aperture setting are inversely proportional. Therefore the larger the aperture of a lens, the faster the

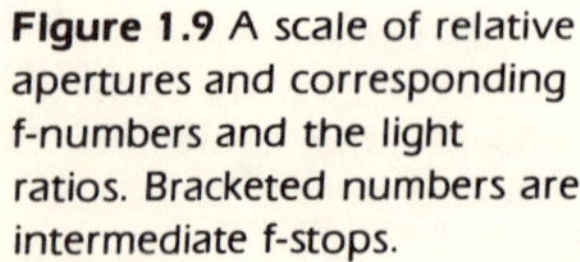

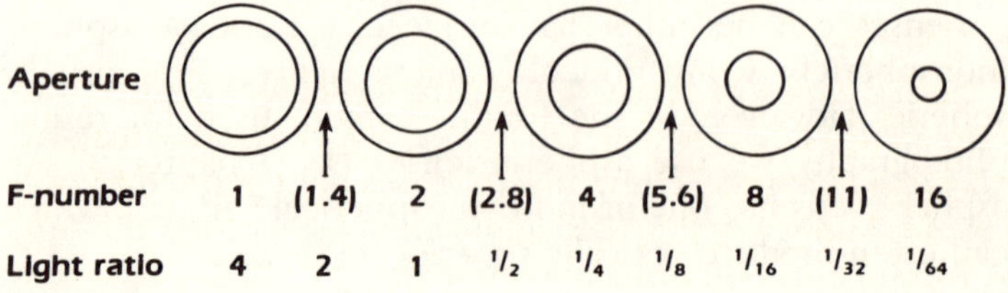

Figure 1.9 A scale of relative apertures and corresponding f-numbers and the light ratios. Bracketed numbers are intermediate f-stops.

shutter speed can be set on the camera body. Using this faster shutter speed setting allows the film to freeze movement in low light situations.

The compromise the photographer makes when using a large aperture is a reduction in depth of field of the subject being photographed. Depth of field is the distance between the closest and farthest objects in a photograph that appear on the film to be in sharp focus. Three things affect depth of field: aperture setting, which increases depth of field as the aperture is stopped down to smaller and smaller diameter settings; the focal length of the lens, depth of field decreasing as focal length increases; and the distance from the lens to the subject, as one moves the lens further away from the film plane and increases magnification, depth of field constricts. With certain ophthalmic cameras (slit lamp and retinal cameras) the angle of view is changed with a magnification changer, which adds supplementary lenses to the principal optical objective lens to increase or decrease image size in the eyepiece and on the film. In all cases the higher the magnification, the smaller the depth of field.

Lenses suffer from manufacturing and physical limitations, called **lens aberrations.** One common aberration is: spherical aberration, which is the tendency of a lens to fail to bring parallel light rays to a common principal focus. The human eye can also suffer this deficiency—astigmatism. Smaller apertures reduce this defect. There are two types of chromatic aberration. In longitudinal, which is a variation in focal length corresponding to wavelengths of light, different colors come to sharp focus at different points on a lens' nodal axis affecting the entire image. Lateral aberration is a variation in magnification with wavelength, affecting the outer edges of images. Lateral aberration is most noticeable at higher magnifications, especially in photomicrography. All lenses are manufactured to produce the best correcting compromise to reduce these defects.

The designation of various types of camera lenses is related to the focal length of the lens. Focal length is the distance from the lens to the plane of focus when the lens has been focused at infinity. Based on the camera format the standard lens is the normal focal length most equivalent to that of the diagonal measure of the film size. *Zoom* lenses are adjustable focal length lenses, ranging either from wide angle to telephoto (35mm–105mm) or short telephoto to long telephoto (70mm–200mm). Zoom lenses are lenses of many focal lengths.

Special types of lenses for enlarging images beyond the scale of life (1:1), called **macro** lenses, will be discussed in the following chapters. These macro lenses are designed to perform best optically at 1:10 magnification rather than at infinity. Most forms of ophthalmic photography use macro lenses

Normal, when applied to camera lenses, means at the same relative magnification as seen by the human eye. The angle of view relates to magnification directly when defining normal. Optically a camera with a normal lens restricts angle of view (or angle of coverage) to approximately 50 degrees. The human eye sees peripherally a greater angle of view, but the area of good definition around fixation is from 30 degrees to 50 degrees. While a film image taken with a normal lens appears smaller, the normal linear perspective the eye sees daily is best reproduced with a lens of this focal length. The larger the camera film format, the longer the normal lens' focal length.

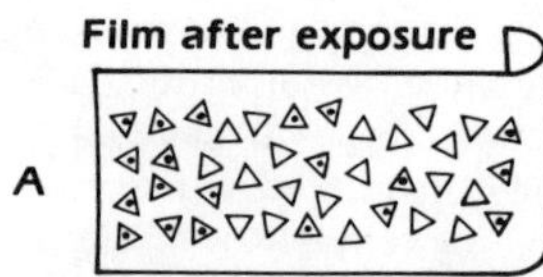

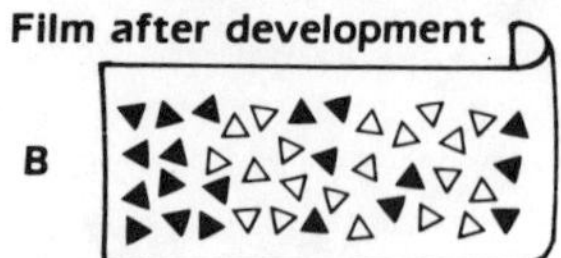

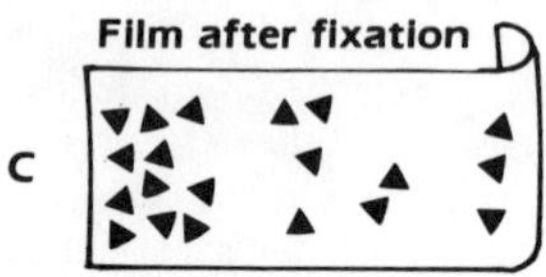

Figure 1.10 A cross-section of a sheet of black-and-white film emulsion
A) ▲ = light struck silver
Δ = unexposed silver
B) ▲ = developed silver
Δ = undeveloped silver
C) ▲ = developed silver.
Unexposed, undeveloped silver is gone.

to make images as most ophthalmic photo images render detail larger than life.

All lenses can be used with a variety of filters to manipulate or correct problems inherent in the subject, the lens being used, or both. Filters can also be used to manipulate or alter light passing through lenses to highlight various aspects of subjects being photographed. Most conventional lenses have screw mounts in front lens surface allowing various filters to be placed between subject and lens.

Film

The third component of a photographic system is the light sensitized material for recording images—the film. The light-sensitized chemical used in most films is silver. Silver is mixed with halogen elements and suspended in gelatin. This dispersion of light-sensitive silver halides is called an **emulsion** (Figure 1.10). That silver is sensitive to light is the key point in understanding the construction and use of film.

History

Silver was discovered to be light sensitive by a German scientist, Johan Heinrich Schultz, in 1725. Schultz left a jar of chalk in silver nitrate on the ledge of his studio in the sun one morning. The silver compound, initially white, he noticed, turned black after this solar exposure. When the silver nitrate was removed from the window sill, it returned to its original white state. In 1757 in Italy another scientist, Giovanni Beccaria, independently demonstrated that light turned silver chloride blue-violet. As time passed and communications improved, the knowledge of silver nitrate's light sensitivity became commonly known. Silver mixed with nitrates suspended in a support material collodion was spread on paper and leather by Thomas Wedgewood in the early 1800s, and silhouettes were made on these treated materials. Silver nitrate paper was also placed in a camera obscura (the first camera) to attempt to form permanent images. The unresolved problem was how to "fix" this chemical reaction so the image would remain permanent. Wedgewood died before solving this problem. He missed the opportunity to father photography.

The first individual to solve the fixation dilemma was a Frenchman, Jospeh-Nicephore Niepce. Looking for a means of making lithographs, and familiar with silver nitrate sensitivity, Niepce used nitric acid to fix his images. His film emulsion, though, the silver was so insensitive that his (and the world's) first true photograph, taken in 1826, required an eight-hour exposure. The next year Niepce met Louis Daguerre, with whom he formed a partnership. In that same year, Niepce went to London to report his work to the Royal Society, who rejected it because he would not explain how it worked. After Niepce's death in 1833, Daguerre developed his patented (1841) method of forming silvered copper plates sensitized with iodine vapors, which were then developed in mercury vapors and fixed in a hot solution of cooking salt—the resulting image was called a Daguerrotype.

At the same time, in England, William Henry Fox Talbot began his own experimentations, treating paper with silver chloride, exposing it, then fixing it in common salt. His report in 1839 to the Royal Society stirred the interest of Sir John Herschel, the astronomer. Herschel wrote to Talbot describing Talbot's process as "photography." Herschel further suggested that Talbot use sodium thiosulfate (hypo) as a fixative agent. Hypo worked. The final piece of the puzzle was uncovered. Talbot's "photographic" process became the film development process we know today.

Initially all film images were black and white. Exposure of film to light rendered a "negative" plate in which black or dark subject areas were rendered as light tones on the film, and white or light areas rendered as dark tones. A second procedure, called printing, was necessary to reverse the pictoral tones of such a negative back to a positive (white as white, black as black) image of the original subject. The negative, however, could be used to produce as many positive images as desired. This process continues to this day.

In 1879, George Eastman of Rochester began manufacturing film plates. In 1888 he introduced a camera, "the Kodak," loaded with a gelatin-based emulsion mounted on transparent flexible film. Roll film was born (and so was Eastman Kodak, Inc.). Black-and-white film became the standard for 50 years in photography; though work on developing color films had begun as early as 1809. Color films were introduced commercially in the mid-to-late 1930s. Two types of color films were developed; the color negative emulsion to make positive color prints, and the color slide transparency, to make positive projectable images. Of the two, slide transparencies are more conventionally used in ophthalmic photography, along with black-and-white negative films.

The normal human eye contains millions of cones in the retina. Color film is like this component of the eye's inner lining. The cones act as color receptors. They are concentrated in the area of our clearest central vision, the fovea. Cones are sensitive to red, blue, and green light radiation. Normal eyes are balanced for daylight full spectrum sensitivity. Color negative films operate essentially the same way. They contain silver-sensitive crystals mixed with three separate dye

The human eye has its own film, the neural sensory retina. It is a multilayered clear neural tissue responsible for converting a percentage of the light energy entering the eye into chemical impulses. These impulses are transmitted via the optic nerve to the brain to produce sight. The sensory retina, being neural brain tissue, is incapable of regeneration once damaged by aging, disease, or accident. The optic nerve is also the only nerve in the body we can see (and photograph). The sensory retina acts as an integrated chip in a computer, constantly recording, transmitting, and then erasing the images that fall upon it. The receptors of the sensory retina are of two types: rods, which separate light from dark, and measure and track movement; and cones, which resolve detail for visual acuity and produce color vision.

layers, each sensitive to either red, green, or blue, which combine when printed or projected to reproduce color. Different film emulsions require specific color development techniques.

Characteristics

All films exhibit certain common characteristics. They are:

Film Speed

Film speed is the sensitivity of a specific film emulsion when exposed to light. The International Standards Organization (ISO) has set a method of rating the speed of photographic materials. The range is from 1 to 3200. This geometrically progressive scale, like time settings on a shutter dial, doubles. Thus a film rated 400 ISO is four times as sensitive as a film rated 100 ISO and requires 1/4 the amount of exposure required by the second to render a similarly lit subject. In certain low-light situations increased film speed makes correct exposure possible. ISO was previously referred to as ASA (American Standards Association).

Grain

Resolution properties of film are measured in line pairs per millimeter. Usually, lower ISO films have greater ability to resolve detail. Both lenses and photographic materials have resolving power.

To test resolution, a target of progressively smaller adjacent light and dark lines is photographed, and the smallest pair of lines distinguishable is determined.

Grain is the size of silver specks in the film emulsion. Film speed is related to silver grain size in the fim. The silver specks in the emulsion vary in size, becoming large and larger as ISO increases. Larger grain reduces image sharpness and resolution of detail. A slow film, such as a 25 ISO color slide film, will have very fine specks of silver, hence very high resolution of images. A fast film, such as a 400 ISO black-and-white negative emulsion, will have various sized silver specks. While the 400 ISO film is 16 times more sensitive to light than the 25 ISO film, its grain sharpness will be greatly reduced, producing less detailed images due to the large silver specks in the emulsion.

Contrast Index

Contrast index is another characteristic of film. Contrast is the variation between highlight and shadow areas rendered in a photographic subject. Contrast describes the capability of film to record these values—white through gray to black. High contrast films record fewer values, mostly the elements that are either black or white. Normal contrast films record a full range of values. Chemical developers can be used to alter the contrast of films.

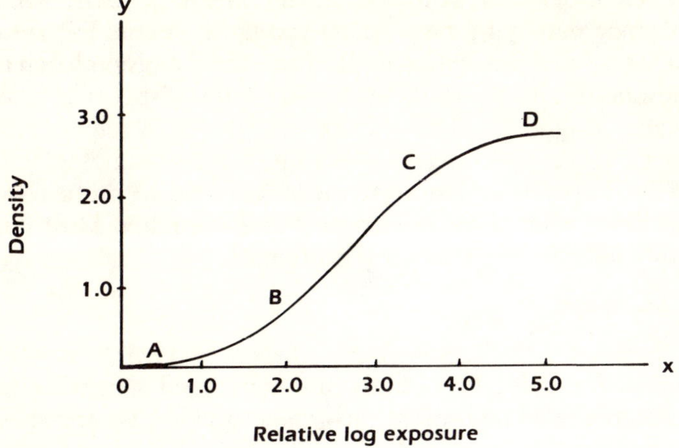

Figure 1.11 The characteristic curve of a negative film. The x-axis represents a logarithm of light exposure. Each unit is 10x the number to its left. The y-axis is a measure of silver density of the film relative to light exposure. **A** is base film density (minimal exposure). **BC** is correct exposure range. **D** is the shoulder—too much exposure.

Density

Density is the physical measure of silver left in the film emulsion after development and fixing in any given area on a piece of film (Figure 1.11). The characteristic curve shown in the figure is a graph of a typical black-and-white negative film. Density is recorded on a developed photo negative material (y-axis) relative to a logarithm of the amount of exposure of light striking that material (x-axis). As more light strikes the film, more density occurs. The slope of the curve is the contrast index of the particular film charted. A steeper slope indicates greater variation between dark and light densities.

The science of *sensitometry* is the measuring and recording of the light sensitivity of a given film. For our purposes, know that a faster speed film has larger grain structure and a smaller slope, that is, less variation in the difference between black and white. Ophthalmic photo instruments, with many lens systems and filters that lose light due to internal reflections, often need high speed films to record the image. Increased grain and the consequent decreased resolution are the price of recording any detail on "fast" film. With positive color slide films the characteristic curve is reversed. Density is erased in development, so the curve drops from the top of the y-axis down and right toward the x-axis. Consult a book on sensitometry for more information (see bibliography).

Color Balance

Color films have specific color balances in each batch of emulsion manufactured. Film is manufactured in large sheets, or batches. The film is cut, sprockets are added, and the film is placed in cannisters. Different batches of the same film type may not render colors exactly the same. Filtration can alter this balance to match closely one emulsion batch to another, but in the practical clinical lab this disparity in color balance is ignored. Critical color work demands require consistent color matching so users buy large volumes of one emulsion batch and store it in refrigerators to protect the film from color shifts due to heat and humidity. Most film boxes indicate the film's batch number.

Types of Films

The following is a list of films commonly used in ophthalmic photography with notes on each one's specific characteristics:

Black-and-White Films

Black-and-white films are usually negative—emulsions in which subject dark tones are rendered light on film and light tones rendered dark. The resulting images contain only tones of gray. ISOs range from 1 to 3200. ISO 400 black-and-white film is used most commonly to create original ophthalmic images. Many other kinds of black-and-white films and papers are used to reverse these negatives to positives for viewing (Figure 1.12).

Color Slide Films

Color slide films are color transparency materials used to produce positive color images, usually in 35mm format. These films, ranging in ISO from 25 to 400 are available in 24- or 36-exposure rolls. When developed, these films are mounted in 2×2 inch cardboard mounts. The positive images are viewed on light boxes, or by projection on a screen. Slide films balanced for daylight are designed to record as accurately as possible the colors of the subject as seen by the photographer's eye—given normal color vision. Slide film exposed with electronic flash is much used in ophthalmic photography.

Color Negative Films

Color negative films are negative materials, containing three black-and-white emulsions mixed with separate color dyes that reverse subject tones on the film in the camera when a picture is taken. The developed negative is then reversed onto color photographic paper to create a positive print. Color negative emulsions usually range in ISO from 100 to 1000. Color negative films have less resolution than color slide

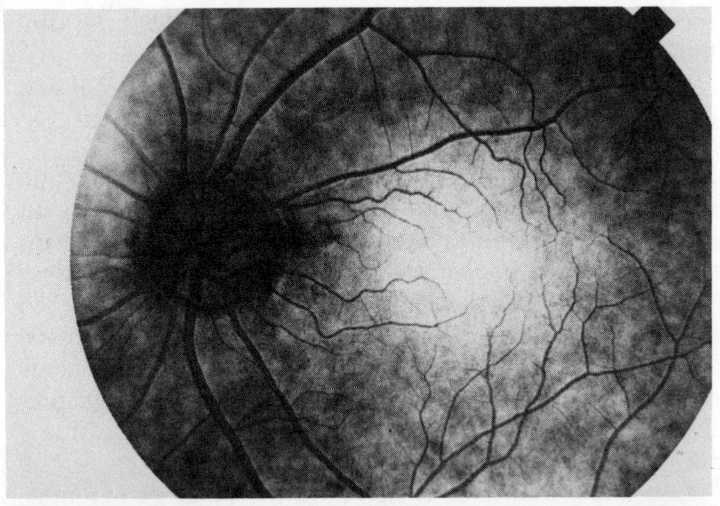

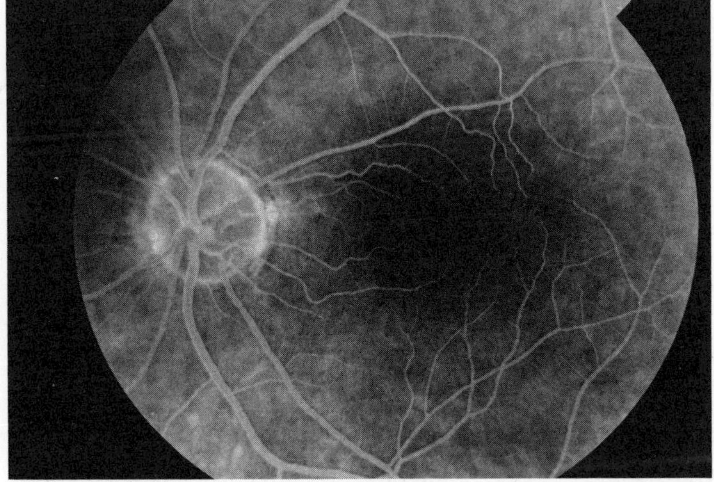

Figure 1.12 The same image as a negative (top) and a positive print (bottom).

films, and are consequently less used in ophthalmic photography.

Polaroid "Instant" Films

Instant films are manufactured with a developing agent incorporated in the film emulsion or in a package adjacent to the film sheet. When a Polaroid sheet film exits the Polaroid film back, rollers break, release and spread these chemicals over the film emulsion. Development occurs in one or more minutes. Polaroid emulsions are available in color or black and white in a variety of ISOs and film sheet sizes.

Some types of Polaroid sheet film produce a negative as well as an instant positive print. The resolution of these films is not always equal to color transparency films. Polaroid instant films are very useful for photographic documentation, patient education, and for training individuals to use ophthalmic photographic instruments.

Autoprocess 35mm Films

This new generation of Polaroid 35mm format color and black-and-white films incorporates a developing/fixing agent in the film emulsion. Polaroid provides a developer kit with each roll of film. A separate film processing unit is necessary to match film and developing kit for processing exposed ages. Film images (all positive transparencies) can be developed dry to dry in under four minutes. The unique emulsion characteristics of these films necessary to make the process work reduce image resolution. When rapid processing is necessary, these films are very useful.

Check any film store to see the wide range of manufacturers producing film, and the varieties of films available. Read the enclosed data sheet to learn more about each film. Ophthalmic photographic camera manufacturers provide guides to the specific ISO of films necessary in each respective instrument. Check for specific applications. As a first resort, check the manual.

Film Development

The fourth component of photography is chemical film development. Development makes the invisible (latent) image on the film visible. Each film type requires different chemical steps to return the silver in the emulsion to its original metallic state, and render the film nonlight sensitive. These development procedures are simpler for black-and-white films. For color slide films the outside processing lab is more consistent and convenient. Black-and-white film development is discussed in Chapter 8.

Chapters 2–7 discuss the methods of correctly exposing film so that when development is complete the pictures taken will be the best results obtainable.

Summary

Light moving through space can be captured in a box on a light-sensitive material. That light-sensitive material can then be removed and processed to render permanent the captured light. Or—we can use a camera loaded with film to take a picture. We then develop (and sometimes) print that film to make a photograph.

CHAPTER 2

External Photography

by J. Michael Coppinger

The first area to examine in ophthalmic photography is the most general and elementary—external photography. Using the camera and film discussed in Chapter One, we perform external photography every time we take a photograph. The degree of magnification and the area of subject to be covered determine the specific equipment to choose for any particular photograph.

The ophthalmologist requesting external documentary photography will usually restrict the subject area to a full face portrait, pictures of both eyes, or one eye at low and high magnification (Figure 2.1).

This range of magnification is easily photographed with a 35mm format camera and the appropriate lens. As range of magnification increases, the designation of the type of photography changes.

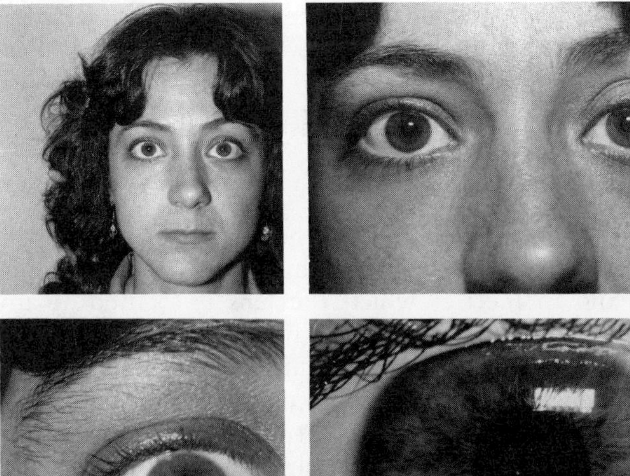

Figure 2.1 An external photo sequence demonstrating full face external at 1:10 (top left), bilateral at 1:4 (top right), orbital at 1:3 (bottom left), and life size at 1:1 (bottom right).

Standard views in external eye photography can be categorized by subject. Normal photo requests will be for full head and shoulders, full face forward, full face profile left and right, both eyes, one eye orbit included, one eye life size, and one eye at 2x magnification.

Type of photography	Magnification range
General photography	Infinity to $\frac{1}{10}$x (1:10)
Close-up photography	$\frac{1}{10}$x to 1x (life-size)
Life-size photography	1:1 (1x)
Photomacrography	1x to 10x (10:1)
Photomicrography	10x to 2000x

Of these five, only photomicrography is outside the range of "external" photography.

Magnification

Magnification is defined as the process of making larger, as in an image compared with an object.

$$\text{Magnification} = \frac{\text{Image Size}}{\text{Object Size}}$$

Optically in the scale of reproduction even though a lens may image an object at $\frac{1}{10}$ its size on the film this is still considered magnification.

Magnification can also be defined mathematically and computed. Focus and magnification are directly related to the distance between the lens and the film plane. If we focus on an object in the foreground, the camera lens is rotated away from the film plane toward the subject to refocus the object on the film. This extension of the lens increases the image size on the film. If we divide the distance of the extension between lens and film in the camera by the focal length of the particular lens we are using we have the mathematical magnification.

$$\text{Magnification} = \frac{\text{Extension Distance} < \text{Lens} < \text{Camera}}{\text{Focal Length of Same Lens}}$$

Camera lenses, for user convenience, often display on the lens focus housing scales that indicate the distance (in meters and in feet) at which the lens is focused at any particular extension. A second numerical scale on this housing indicates the corresponding magnification ratio of focused image relative to the focus distance scale (Figure 2.2). Thus a 55mm lens focused at 2.5 feet produces a magnification ratio of 1:10. Close up photography ($\frac{1}{10}$x to 1x) requires a special camera lens designed to focus closer than 2.5 feet. The two scales on the lens continue to higher magnification ratios as the lens moves closer to the object and further from the film plane. For example, a 55mm close up lens focused on an object at 35cm from the lens has a magnification of approximately 1:4 on the film.

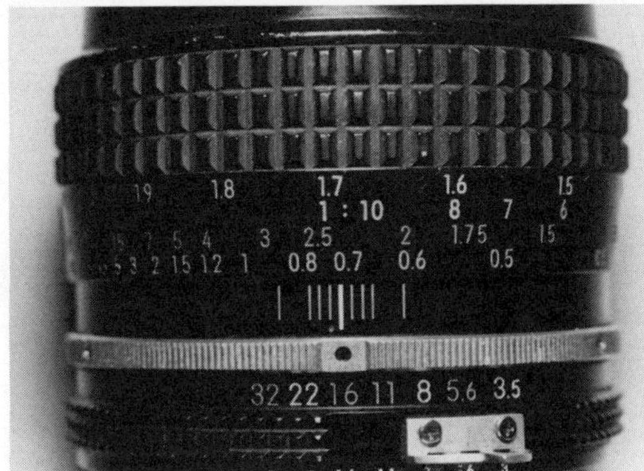

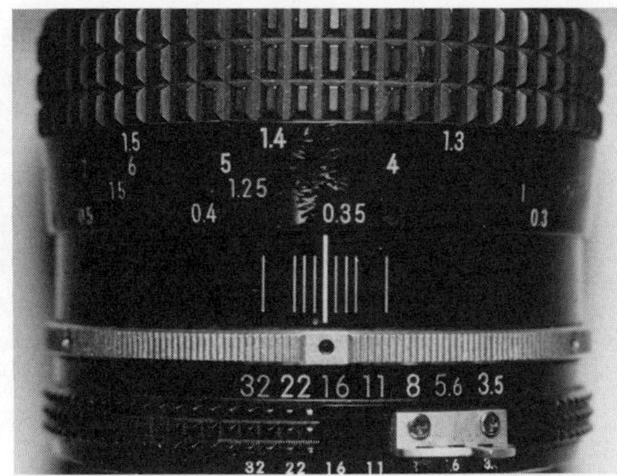

Figure 2.2 A 55mm micro Nikor lens. The lowest set of numbers, 32–3.5, represent apertures. The aperture selected is f-16 in both photos. The scales above the scored lines represent range of focus (depth of field). The next higher numeric scales are meters, then feet. The 1:10 scale represents magnification on the film in the camera. This lens is focused at 2.5 feet (.7 cm) creating a 1:10 magnification on film (left). This lens is focused at 1.2 feet (.35 cm) creating a 1:3.5 magnification on film (right).

To increase magnification to life size (1:1) and beyond, more specialized lenses, extension tubes, or bellows must be added to the camera lens system. The camera lens at these degrees of magnification moves further from the film plane, and closer to the subject. This increased distance from lens to film reduces the amount of light reaching the film. If the lens distance is doubled, the light intensity on the film is quartered. Thus, the indicated aperture has changed though the f stop aperture setting remains the same on the lens housing.

The effective aperture being used is actually ¼ (or two f-stops) less than the f-stop set on the lens. Remember a higher numbered f-stop indicates a decrease in the amount of light passing through the lens. Therefore, creating an image magnification of 1:2 (or 2x) moves the lens further from the film and requires an increase in exposure to compensate for the reduced amount of light passing through the lens to the film. We can calculate this effective aperture by multiplying the aperture on the lens by the sum of magnification plus a constant of one f-stop. Therefore:

Effective Aperture = Aperture on Lens (Magnification + 1)

$$A_E = A_1 \ (M+1)$$

So for given aperture f8 and a magnification of 2x:

$$A_E = f8\,(2 + 1)$$

$$A_E = f24$$

F24 is approximately 2 f-stops smaller than f8 so increase exposure by more than 2 f-stops (= 4× times more exposure) to render a useful image on film. The following exposure scale correlates magnification relative to aperture correction required. This scale applies to all focal length lenses used in external photography. Many lens manufacturers provide such a chart with the lens purchased.

While computing magnification by formula is always possible, in clinical practice framing the subject to fill the viewfinder is all that is required. Tests should always be done to determine effective aperture relative to flash exposure for all pictures with magnifications greater than life size. To preserve depth of field always increase flash output and work at small aperture settings. Use of specific magnifications (1:1, 2:1) will facilitate obtaining correct consistent and comparable results.

Magnification of image	Aperture correction required in f stops
.1	.28
.5	1.17
1.0	2.00
1.5	2.67
2.0	3.17
2.5	3.61
3.0	4.00
3.5	4.34
4.0	4.64

We will return to effective aperture when discussing photomacrography techniques.

Selecting Equipment

Many camera manufacturers offer similar camera bodies and lenses for use to take external to "macro" photographs. We will consider the components only generically.

Camera Body Format

The optimal single camera lens combination for versatile external photography is a 35mm single lens reflex camera, a 105mm macro lens with a bellows or extension tubes, and a single flash unit that can operate on and off-the camera. When the flash is not mounted on the camera, but hand held, make sure to have a power cord connection (PC cord) long enough to freely move to any desired position to direct the flash onto the subject from any desired angle.

The most common and useful film/camera format is 35mm, usually of the single lens reflex (SLR) variety. To review, a single lens reflex camera uses one lens for focusing as well as exposure. When the shutter release is fired, the reflex mirror lifts out of the light path to the film plane to allow the image to be recorded on film.

The 35mm SLR cameras display in the viewfinder the same image magnification being recorded on the film. Lenses are easily interchanged on these camera bodies. New features on some camera systems include "on the film plane" metering for correct automatic exposure regardless of the lens being used. Small computer microchips in the camera body compute exposures, even when the camera is connected to electronic flash devices. These TTL (through the lens) systems are "dedicated", that is, they work automatically when coupled with lens and flash unit of like design. Such automatic systems simplify photography, but they sometimes oversimplify and fail to expose correctly. Always test a new system before using it with patients.

Camera Lenses

Select two good lenses for use, one of short focal length (55mm) and one of long (105mm). These should be "macro" or "micro" lenses made to focus at close distances. The 55mm lens works for general photography from infinity to $^1/_{10}$x and close up photography $^1/_{10}$x to .5x. **Extension rings**

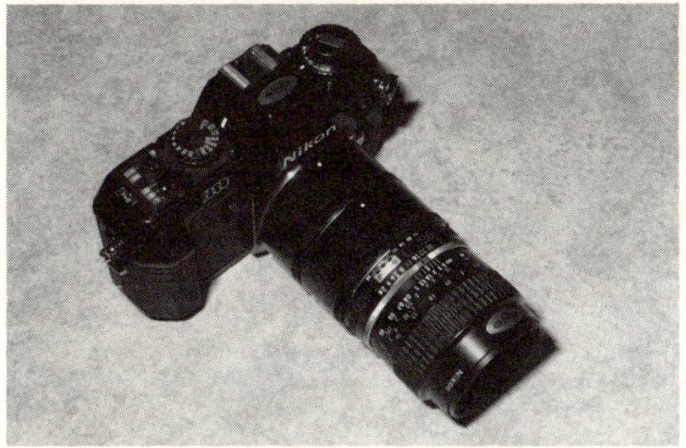

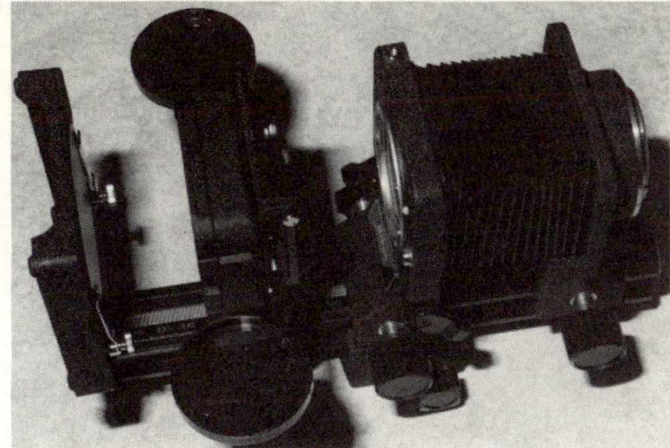

Figure 2.3 Two methods of increasing image magnification: A 35mm camera with two extension rings between the lens and camera body (left). A bellows attachment, in this case part of a slide duplicator. For external photography an independent bellows is recommended for easy magnification changes (right).

or bellows can be added between lens and camera body to increase magnification to life size (1:1) and greater (Figure 2.3). Some macro lenses can be reversed and mounted backwards on the camera body to increase magnification. These reversible lenses are optically designed to form a focused image when mounted backward. A reversing ring is screwed onto the front of the lens; the outside of this reversing ring has a lens mount. The lens is then mounted backward on the camera body. When reversed, the lens acts as a magnifier and increases image size (up to 3:1).

The 55mm lens requires a short working distance between camera and patient. For this reason, many photographers prefer a 105mm "macro" lens. This close focus lens moves the camera position further from the subject. It also corrects the barrel distortion induced by shorter working distances, that is, the bowing distortion of the edges of the image. The increase in working distance, from camera to patient, permits more lighting control, reduces corneal reflections, and produces more aesthetically pleasing pictures. A longer focal length is desirable when doing motility studies, such as, documenting the nine standard fields of gaze required for strabismus photography (Figure 2.4). Motility studies are per-

Figure 2.4 The nine standard fields of gaze photographed to record ocular muscle deviations: up right (1), up center (2), up left (3), right (4), center (5), left (6), down right (7), down center (8), down left (9).

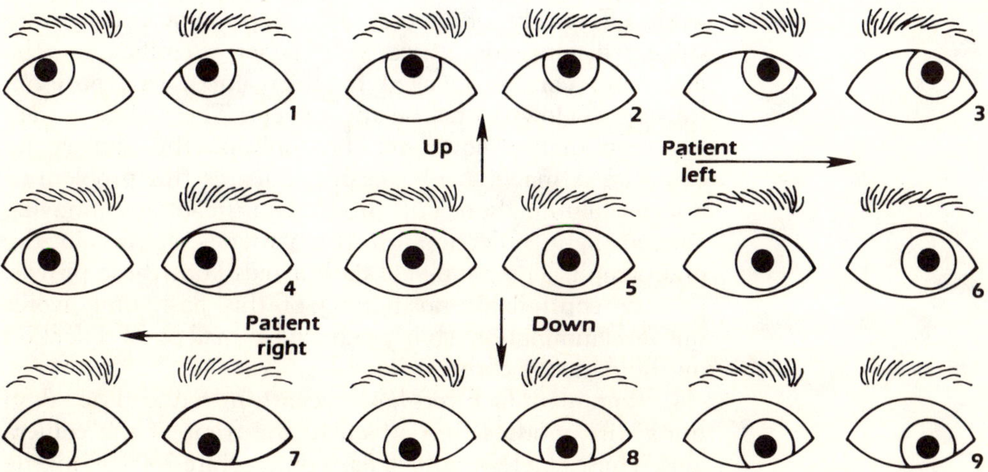

formed to document ocular muscle disorders, deviations of gaze and other conditions affecting fixation and convergence.

Some camera lenses accept a Teleconverter, an extension ring with an optical magnifier placed between the lens and camera. The teleconverter doubles the focal length of the lens, thus doubling the image magnification in the viewfinder and on the film. With a teleconverter, a 50mm focal length lens becomes a 100mm focal length lens. These teleconverters, while useful, have two drawbacks. First, they reduce light in the viewfinder for focusing. Second, teleconverters cut relative aperture by one full stop. For example, f8 on the aperture ring is f11 on the film plane, and requires a doubling of exposure time or flash output to correctly record an image.

The supplementary magnifying devices (bellows, extension tubes, teleconverters) can often decouple the automatic exposure features of the dedicated camera system. Check your camera manual to insure proper use of these devices with electronic flash.

Flash Units for Lighting

While many special flash units have been developed for external ophthalmic photography, the use of even the simplest of manual electronic flash units will work effectively in general in close up and macro photography.

Many flash units are made specially for "close up" lenses. The most common are: 1) standard flash units, which can be mounted on top of the camera body or hand held; ring flashes that attach to the front of the camera lens; and rotating flash units, which can be positioned manually by the photographer to illuminate from any angle the photographer chooses (Figure 2.5). Each type of flash unit has advantages and disadvantages.

The positioning of the flash on top of the camera body works effectively for general photography but as camera to subject distance decreases with higher magnification, the flash unit can be blocked by the camera lens position, causing shadows to fall on the subject. These shadows are not seen in the viewfinder, but only on the film as the exposure is made. A ring flash eliminates this problem of uneven illumination but produces instead an annoying circular light reflection on the patient's cornea in the photograph. The hand-held flash avoids both these pitfalls. Correct controllable positioning of this flash unit avoids uneven illumination while producing a small point reflection on the patient's cornea.

Certain manufacturers have recently introduced ring flash units with mounts that attach to the front of the camera lens. These single or double flash units rotate 360° about the

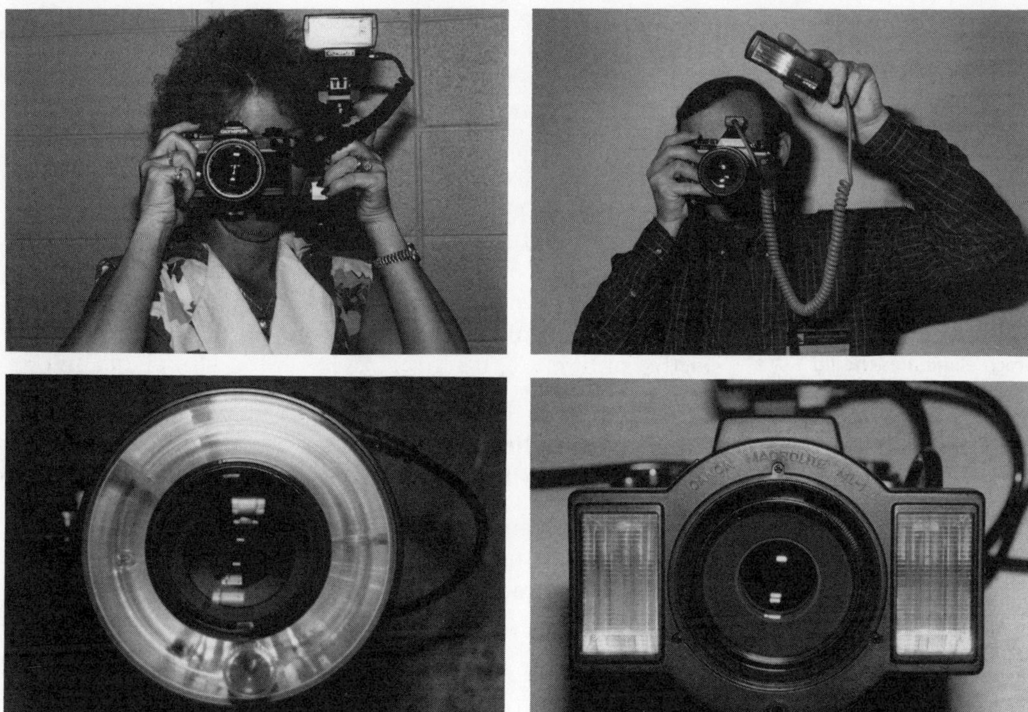

Figure 2.5 Different methods of flash devices used in external photography: Bracket mounted flash unit (top left). Hand-held flash unit (top right). Lens mounted ring flash (bottom left). Rotating flash unit (bottom right).

lens, and allow the photographer to select the best position to place the flash to prevent obscuring the pathology change with a flash reflex (Figure 2.5). Some of these newer flash systems are computerized and measure light reflected off the subject through the camera lens (TTL). These systems compute the correct level of flash output necessary to properly illuminate the subject relative to the f-stop selected, and the ISO of the film in the camera. These automatic features also calibrate the effective aperture necessary for increased magnification, saving the photographer much experimentation. The use of a completely manual flash unit requires calculation of effective aperture relative to magnification. To do this, use a roll of film to test exposures with the manual flash unit. Photograph and record, step by step, a bracketed series (successive f-stops) of exposures for various subjects and magnifications—full face, 1:2, 1:1. Review the results. Write a table of correct exposures for each degree of magnification and place this near or on the camera for future reference. Always use the same ISO film used for the test and the same flash placement.

It may be necessary to mask a manual flash unit in order to reduce its light output when working close to a subject. If the flash unit is too bright, an opaque piece of cardboard with a dime size hole in its center can be placed over the flash to reduce light output to workable levels. Conduct a

Lids often interfere with good composition. Holding lids is an art in making good photographs. Fingers and cotton tipped applicators both work effectively. Use the cotton applicator to roll lids up, by placing the cotton end on the orbital margin of the lid and rotating up and out. The lid will roll onto the applicator. Whenever possible use a magnification which eliminates the lid holder from the picture.

second exposure test when introducing or modifying the flash unit with a mask.

However, with the excellent TTL dedicated flash systems available today, using a manual system is rapidly becoming obsolete.

Whether you use a manual system, or a dedicated system, always remember to preset the flash unit to the ISO of the film being used. In dedicated systems, setting the ISO on the camera back will often also set the flash ISO to coincide with that set on the camera back, thus dedicating the system. Check the flash unit manual to confirm the proper way to set the system.

The Five Cardinal Rules of External Eye Photography

Regardless of camera, lens, or magnification chosen, five basic principles should be mastered and applied to make any good photographic images. They are:

Patient Stability

The comfort and stability of the subject will directly affect the photographs. The higher the degree of magnification the smaller the depth of field and the more patient movement will hinder sharp focus. Select a specific area in the office as a "studio." Position the patient on a stool. For 1:2 and greater magnifications stability can best be achieved by mounting a slit lamp chin rest on a small table and placing the patient within it to confine all but lid and eye movements (Fig. 2.5). The chinrest is also useful for ocular motility studies (Fig. 2.4).

Flash Illumination

Minimize patient movement with electronic flash exposures. Such a rapid controlled light source allows one to use smaller apertures (eg. f22) which give greater depth of field in photographs. Flash photography is also less discomforting to the patient.

Reflection Control

The curved surface of the eye's cornea covered with tear film reflects light very strongly. All extraneous room light should be eliminated for exposure. Background shadows can be eliminated by placing a flat black paper or cloth on the wall behind the patient. This will eliminate unwanted

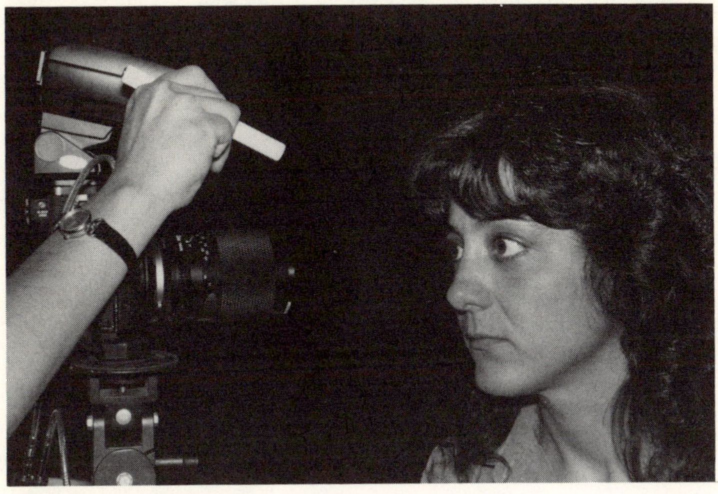

Figure 2.6 Use of a penlight to preview the flash reflex—note the dark background and the camera mounted on a tripod.

subject shadows (Figure 2.6). Use a penlight or tensor lamp to focus the image prior to exposure. Turn this focus light off before taking pictures. Try not to use a room with unshaded windows. Turn off all room lights except the focusing lamp. The windows and room lights will be reflected on the cornea, and in the picture. Try to eliminate all but the flash reflection.

Camera Stability

Buy a tripod and mount the camera on it. (Figure 2.6). The tripod frees both hands for a variety of other tasks. Buy a cable release to allow remote firing of the camera. Hand held photos require a stability for focusing usually impossible for the ophthalmic photographer at higher than 1:10 magnification.

Standardization

Use the same ASA film. Select equipment and perform a series of test exposures at various commonly used scales of magnification. Calibrate the desired useful exposures for each given lighting condition, (i.e., full face, one eye, etc.), and magnification and refer to these exposure calculations when setting up to photograph a patient. This will help prevent exposure errors. Mark images with the degree of magnification selected to allow repetition and comparison of similar subjects photographed over a duration of time (from one sitting to the next).

Make these five rules part of your work method and technique. They will provide ample rewards for the small investment in time, testing and equipment.

The nine standard fields of gaze are photographed in sequence (Figure 2.4). They are up left, up center, up right, right, center left, down left, down center and down right. Use a 100 + mm lens on the camera to avoid lens distortion. The camera should always be the same distance from all patients, the patient's head in a chin rest. This type of photography is done to document ocular muscle deviations, exo- (out) and eso- (in) tropias. Such a series can be done both preoperatively and postoperatively on strabismus patients.

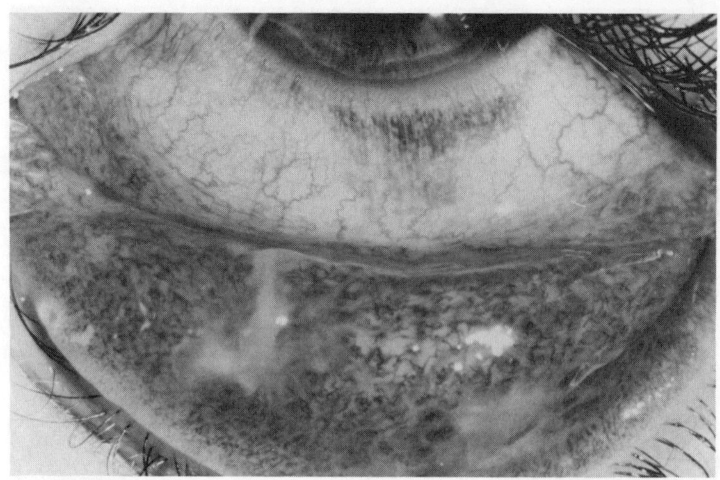

Figure 2.7 Lid holding outside the picture frame.

Step-by-Step Phototechnique

Applying the five cardinal rules previously listed:

1. Position the patient comfortably on a chair or stool in front of a dark background.
2. Insure the camera is loaded, and film ISO is properly set.
3. Check flash synchronization setting (shutter speed).
4. Check the flash unit is properly charged. Use an AC adaptor cord from a wall socket to power the camera whenever possible, rather than rely upon batteries.
5. Mount the camera with cable release on a tripod or similar mount.
6. Turn off all extraneous room lights.
7. Compose the image at the desired magnification in the camera viewfinder. Ensure that if lid holding is necessary the Q-tip or finger holding the lid is outside the picture frame (Figure 2.7).

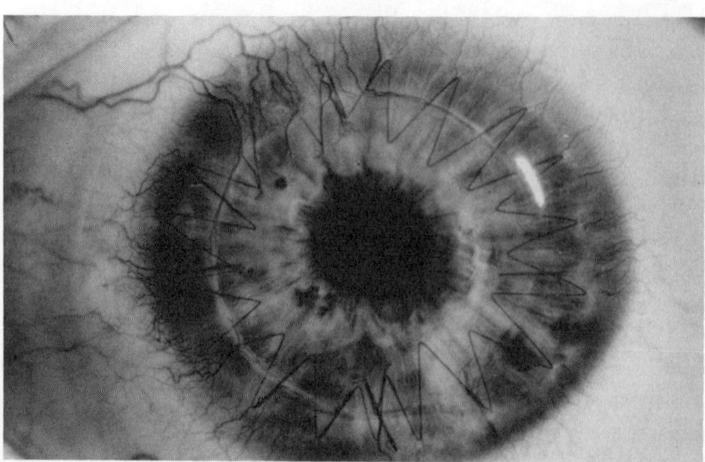

Figure 2.8 Good flash placement to minimize obscuration of pathology change.

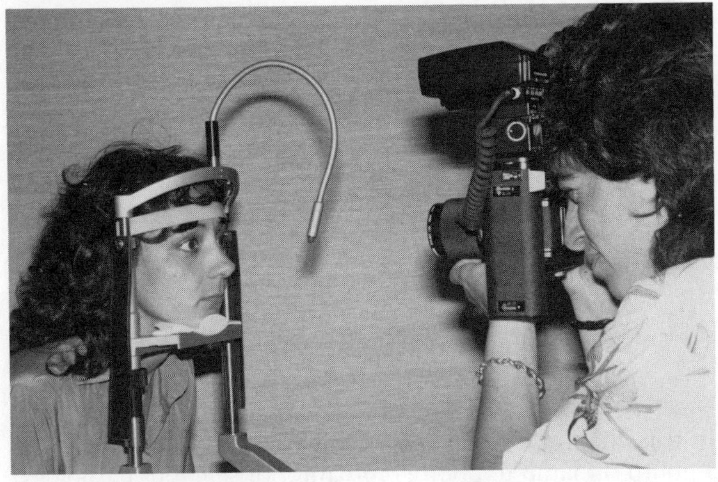

Figure 2.9 Use of a chinrest to stabilize the patient. The chinrest here has an extraneous flexible fixation device which should be removed for binocular photography.

8. Use a penlight or small electric light to illuminate and focus. Direct this light from the same position as the flash while viewing through the eyepiece to observe the flash reflex as it will appear in the picture. Model the light to insure the pathology is not obscured by the flash reflex. Turn the modeling light off before photography (Figure 2.8).
9. At high magnification place the patient's head in a chin rest to reduce motion and blurred focus due to patient movement (Figure 2.9).
10. Select the appropriate f-stop for maximum depth of field in the photo and correct exposure.

here has an extraneous flexible fixation device which should be removed for binocular photography.

11. Position the flash as desired (correct position and exposure have been determined by a controlled exposure test).
12. Expose, wind on, and compose your next image.

Summary

The documentation of external eye disease requires an understanding of the principles of image magnification, close up lens and electronic flash units used with 35mm (or larger format) cameras. Attention should be paid to the comfort and stability of the patient, effective working distance, camera stability, image composition, and standardization of technique for the particular pathology change being photographed.

CHAPTER 3

Slit Lamp Photography

by Mark Maio

In this chapter we will learn the basic techniques for using a photo slit lamp to photograph anterior segment pathology. A thorough review of ophthalmic anatomy is recommended to all slit lamp camera users.

Although slit lamps operate under the same basic principles, there are so many brands that it would be impossible to illustrate the control and operation of each brand of slit lamp camera in a single chapter. The Zeiss photo slit lamp will be used as a model. The discussion is limited to techniques and features common to most currently available photo slit lamps.

Unlike fundus photography, in which knowledge of basic mechanics of camera operation and continued practice result in consistent quality photographs, slit lamp photography presents some unique challenges. The ophthalmic photographer must learn how to use the equipment, recognize normal anterior segment anatomy and anterior pathology, and have the photographic knowledge to record these conditions on film.

This being the case, formal photographic training is a distinct advantage in performing slit lamp photography. Taking a basic course in general photography is highly recommended for ophthalmic medical assistants. Such courses are usually offered at junior colleges, adult education programs, or local photography schools. Understanding how to "see" light and its effect on the film will help one avoid many of the setbacks that beginning slit lamp photographers have to overcome.

The slit lamp biomicroscope, as a photographic instrument, uses focal illumination in the examination of the anterior segment of the eye.

In strictly photographic terms, photography of the anterior segment of the eye can be compared to photographing a small product in a photography studio. In the studio, the photographer uses different lighting techniques, or placements, to best show off a product. For instance, the product might look best when the light is directed in from the front, back, or at a steep angle off to one side. At times the photographer might use a combination of two or three light positions to photograph the product; only by looking at the product and moving the lights can the photographer judge which position or lighting "technique" should be used to do the photograph.

As ophthalmic photographers, we can use this same approach when given the task of using the photo slit lamp to photograph anterior segment pathology. The photo slit lamp with its different light sources and controls becomes our "studio," while the anterior segment pathology becomes our "product." The variable adjustments of the instrument, along with our knowledge of light and how it affects film can then be used to demonstrate a particular type of pathology.

The Slit Lamp

Whether used for clinical examinations or photography, both types of slit lamps share many of the same features.

Common Components

The Slit Lamp Illuminator

The slit lamp illuminator provides the basis around which the rest of the system is built (Figure 3.1). The cornea resembles a watch crystal in its shape and transparent appearance, so visualization requires a special light source; light adjustments possible with the slit lamp illuminator enable the photographer to record fine anterior segment details.

The controls on the slit lamp illuminator allow the photographer to adjust the height, width, or vertical and

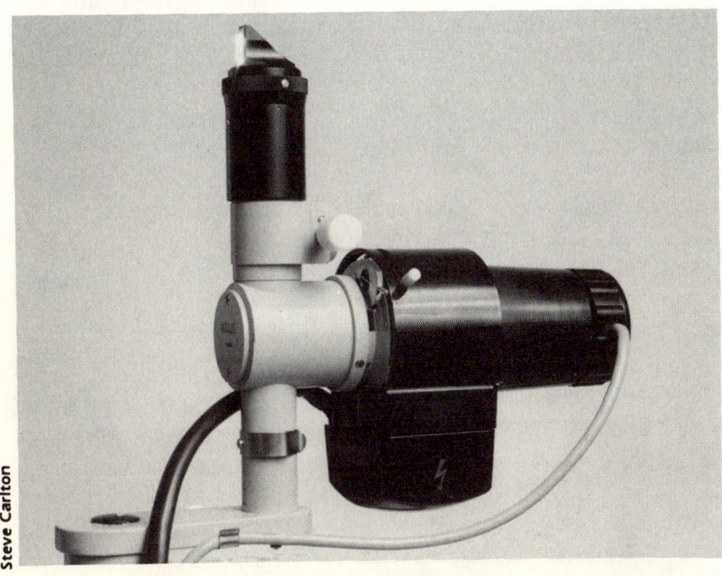

Steve Carlton

Figure 3.1. Slit lamp illuminator.

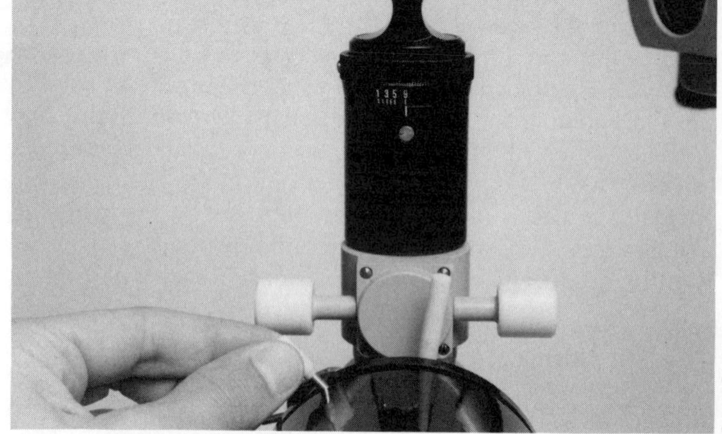

Figure 3.2 Slit beam controls; the short lever controls slit height, the tall lever controls slit width, the two white knobs control the slit beam's right to left position.

horizontal placement of the beam of light (Figure 3.2 and Figures 3.7 through 3.10). This beam of light can vary in size from a tall, thin shaft to a full round circle. The angle at which light enters the eye can also be controlled; the illuminator rotates on a central pivot and this can swing 180° for gross placement of the beam of light on the cornea.

The slit lamp illuminator also has a fine adjustment control to move the light beam in small increments from left to right. When this adjustment is maintained in the central or neutral position, any beam of light coming from the slit illuminator will appear centered and sharply focused when viewed through the optical head of the slit lamp.

One hundred years of developments and modifications preceded the introduction of the slit lamp as we know it today. This instrument couples a separate light house that can be rotated in front of the optical head to direct light from either side of the observation point.

Optical Head

The ability to view changes in the light beam's position is controlled by the optical head of the slit lamp (Figure 3.3). This component of the system provides the photographer

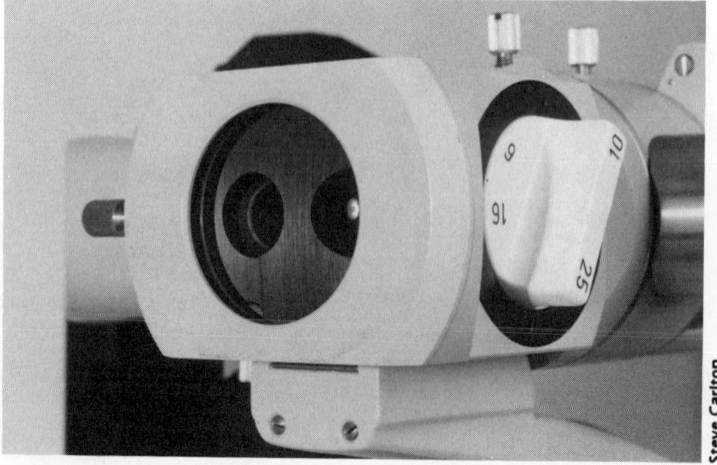

Figure 3.3 Optical head.

with a binocular, magnified, three dimensional view that can be used for examination, or with attachments, for photography (Figure 3.4). The optical head is designed to be parfocal with the slit lamp illuminator; specifically, when the beam of light is in its centered position on the illuminator, an image of that beam will fall into sharp focus at the plane of focus through the optical head. The optical head also swings 180° on the same pivoting point as the slit lamp illuminator. This design allows a focused and centered image of the beam of light, regardless of the angle setting of a component.

Accessories Unique to Photo Slit Lamps

Electronic Flash

Both the clinical exam slit lamp and the photo slit lamp require a source of illumination for viewing. This is usually a small incandescent light bulb controlled by a rheostat that allows the viewing intensity to be increased or decreased. However, while the intensity of this light is high, it is not sufficient for photography.

Photo slit lamps incorporate an electronic flash tube for photography in this same light path. The flash tube is triggered when an exposure is made, and the bright output of light overpowers the viewing light. This is the light that makes the exposure on the film. The amount of light produced is controlled by a calibrated knob on the flash unit's power source. This variable power setting allows a choice of different light outputs.

In addition to the quantity of light produced by the electronic flash, its short duration ($^1/_{1000}$ of a second), stops

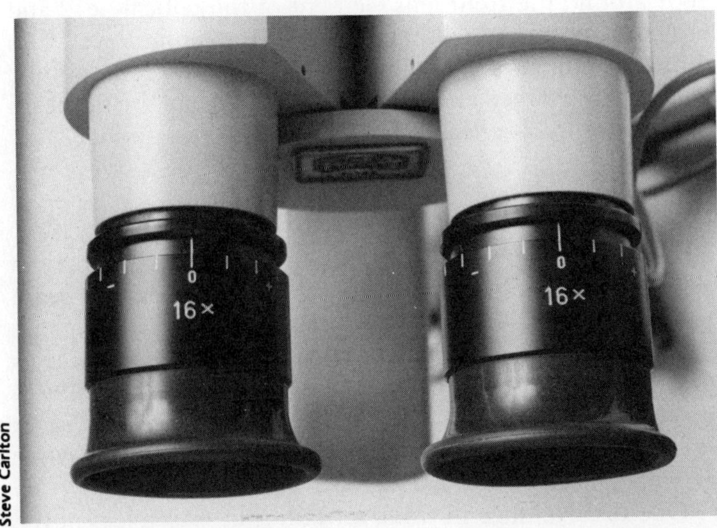

Steve Carlton

Figure 3.4 Binocular eyepieces.

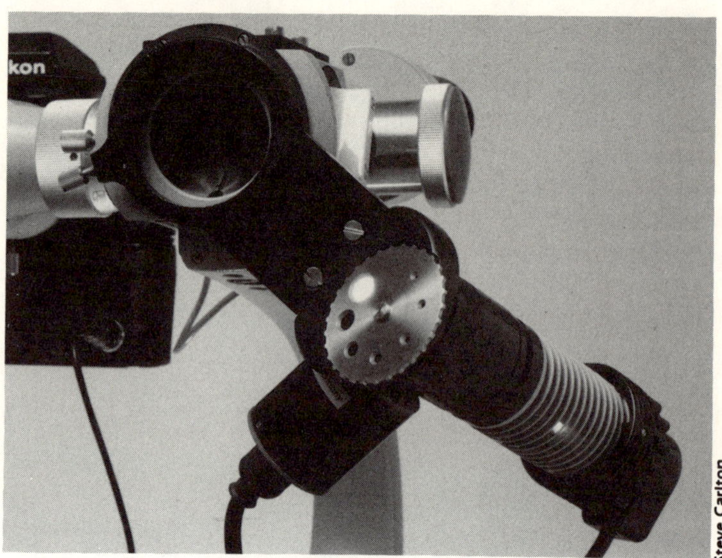

Steve Carlton

Figure 3.5 Diffuse illuminator.

any eye movement during exposure. The "quality" or "color" of the light produced by electronic flash is very similar to daylight, thereby allowing the use of daylight-balanced color slide film.

Background Diffuse Illuminator

Besides having an electronic flash tube in the slit lamp illuminator, most photo slit lamps have an auxillary light source referred to as a background diffuse illuminator (Figure 3.5). Unlike the light of the slit beam, which is focused and controlled, this light source emits a diffuse and scattered light similar to that of a penlight. It can be rotated 360° around the front lens element of the optical head and provides an overall illumination of the entire eye. The diffuse illuminator also contains an electronic flash tube which is discharged along with the flash tube in the slit beam illuminator upon release of the shutter in the camera.

Beam Splitter

The ability to view through the optical head and photograph at the same time is made possible through the use of a beam splitter (Figure 3.6). The beam splitter produces two images with the aid of a combination of prisms. One image is directed to the viewer through the oculars, and the other is diverted to the camera so that the camera "sees" the same image the viewer does. Adjusting lighting techniques while viewing allows you to photograph what you see.

One disadvantage in using a beam splitter is a loss in the amount of light that reaches the oculars. Because examina-

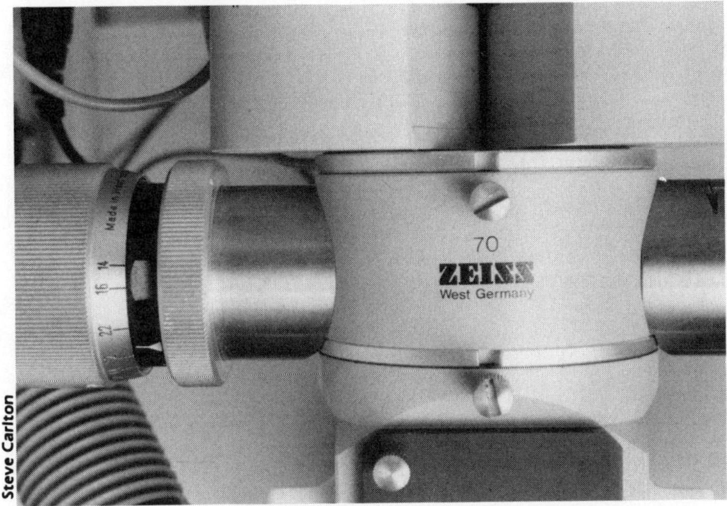

Steve Carlton

Figure 3.6 Beam splitter with photo adaptor.

tion slit lamps do not incorporate beam splitters into their systems, 100% of the light reflected off the subject's eye reaches the oculars. Depending on which type of photo slit lamp is being used, the amount of light reaching the oculars can be reduced to only 15% as a result of the beam splitter's presence. This necessary compromise reduces the amount of fine corneal detail that is visable. It also requires an increase in viewing illumination which may, at times, be very uncomfortable for the patient.

In an effort to compensate for the light reduction, several manufacturers have incorporated a control lever in the beam splitter. This lever allows the beam splitter to be flipped out of the way so that 100% of the viewing light reaches the oculars. At the instant a photograph is to be made, the beam splitter is flipped back into place, and the exposure is made. As a safety measure, the camera will not operate until the beam splitter is in place.

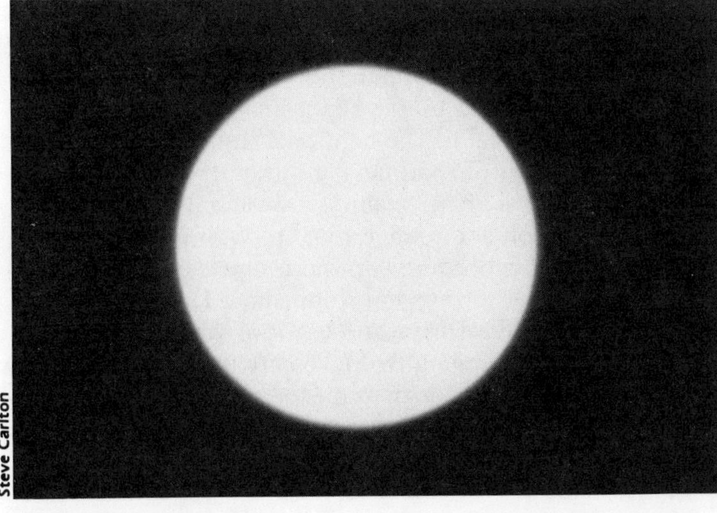

Steve Carlton

Figure 3.7 Slit beam set at full height and width setting.

The Camera Body

In order to record an image on film, photo slit lamps come equipped with a 35mm camera body attached to the beam splitter to perform the task of storing and moving film. Significantly, the image quality is a function of the optics of the photo slit lamp, rather than the 35mm camera used.

Reticule in Eyepiece

Note the step-by-step procedure outlined for setting the ocular reticule on a slit lamp camera. This procedure is necessary with ophthalmic photographic instruments to ensure properly focused images. The image as it will appear on film is viewed through the eyepiece with the reticule—usually the right eyepiece.

A crosshair reticule, similar to that found in a fundus camera, is located in the ocular on the same side of the beam splitter as the camera.

This reticule, properly set, is necessary as a reference point to achieve sharply focused photographs. The accommodative abilities of the photographer's own eye are not noticeable during a clinical examination because the examiner's accommodation creates a focused image. Ignoring the need to nullify accommodation during photography will only result in consistently out-of-focus photographs, because the camera cannot accommodate like the photographer.

To overcome this obstacle, the photographer must establish the correct eyepiece setting to compensate for his or her own refractive error. Obtaining a sharp image of the reticule overlying a focused image of the eye will guarantee sharp photographs. The correct eyepiece setting may be achieved by following these steps:

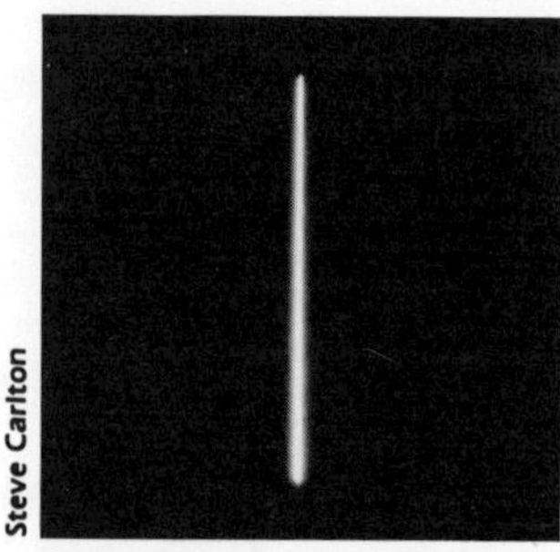
Steve Carlton

Figure 3.8 Thin vertical slit beam.

1. Turn the eyepiece all the way to the maximum plus setting.
2. Tape a piece of white paper to the headrest assembly in front of the photo slit lamp. By placing it close to the front of the lens, and turning on the diffuse illuminator, you should observe a light-colored, unfocused background.
3. Look through the oculars, with your accommodation relaxed, and turn the eyepiece toward the minus side in a slow, continuous motion.
4. Continue turning until a sharp image of the reticule is visualized against the light background. Do not go past the point of sharpness and then try to turn it back until it is sharp again. This will only cause accommodation and render your setting useless.
5. Repeat this procedure two more times, each time recording the setting you stopped at. Take an average of these three settings, and use it as your eyepiece setting for photography. Make sure the other ocular is also positioned for the same setting.

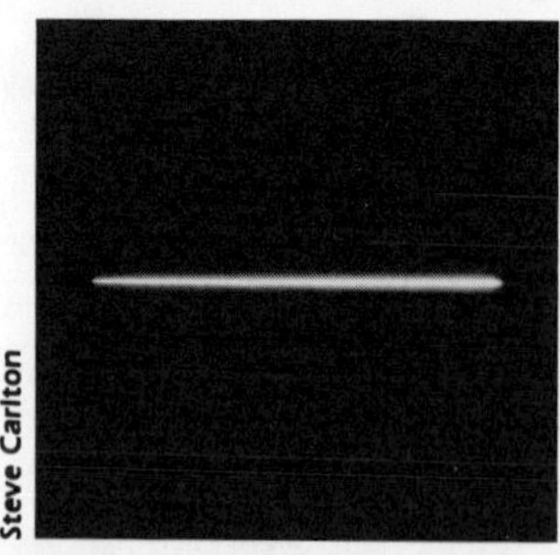
Steve Carlton

Figure 3.9 Thin horizontal slit beam.

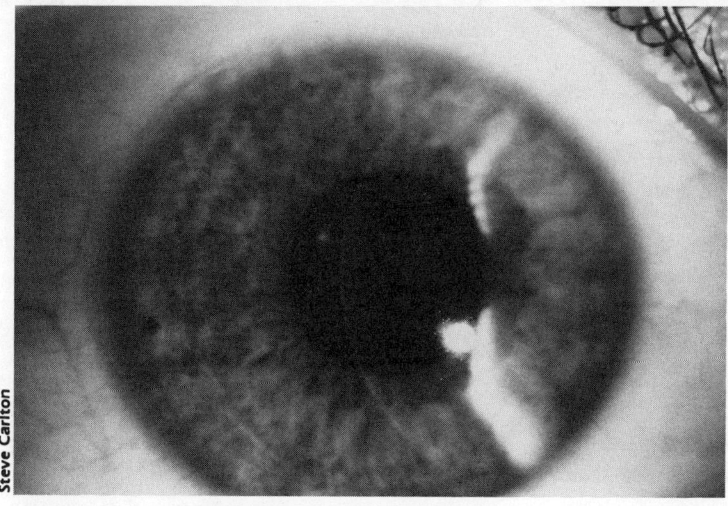
Steve Carlton

Figure 3.10 A thin vertical slit beam projected onto a patient's cornea demonstrating the cross-section effect.

Types of Illumination

Most beginning photographers using the photo slit lamp want a chart recommending lighting techniques for various types of pathology. This might seem easier at first, but it does not force the photographer to think about the effect the light might have on the pathology.

The beginner should learn the basic anterior segment lighting techniques and experiment with them while photographing different types of pathology. As you learn the effect the light has on your "product," you will become better educated in determining lighting choices on the next patient with that dystrophy. However, the presentation of a given dystrophy can vary greatly from one patient to the next, and while one lighting technique might prove adequate in recording the condition in one patient, the appearance of the same dystrophy in another patient could be so radically different that it requires a completely different form of lighting.

Diffuse Illumination

Depending on the type of photo slit lamp being used, diffuse illumination (Figure 3.11) can be accomplished in one of three ways. Most photo slit lamps have a background diffuse illuminator that projects a diffuse light on the eye and allows an overall view of the general condition of the eye. Other photo slit lamps do not come equipped with a background-diffuse illuminator but have a piece of frosted plastic that fits over the top of the slit lamp illuminator.

Diffuse illumination is light spread equally over the entire surface of an object viewed through the biomicroscope.

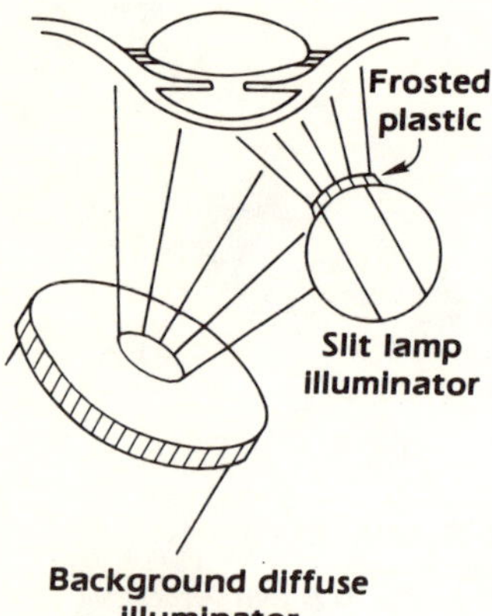

Figure 3.11 Diffuse illumination.

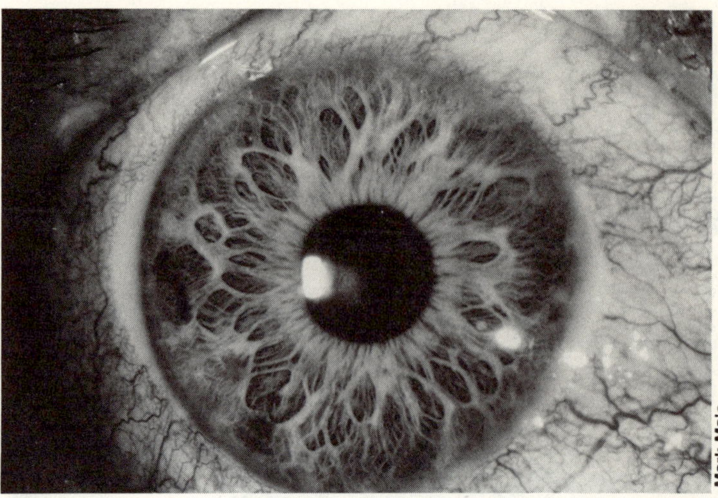

When the slit beam is opened to a full wide circle of light, the plastic diffuses and scatters the light, producing an effect similar to that of the background illuminator. The third option utilizes both the background illuminator and the slit lamp illuminator with diffuser. Having a source of diffuse illumination on either side of the eye produces a balanced and even light across the ocular area.

The technique of using diffuse illumination, although considered the most basic, is also one of the most useful. From an informational standpoint, it is absolutely necessary and should be included on each patient photographed.

Direct Illumination

By varying the type of direct illumination used, the photographer can document the general condition of the eye.

The four basic forms of direct illumination are optical section, optical section with diffuse illumination, broad-beam illumination, and broad-tangential illumination. These four forms of illumination are the most useful means of documenting the general condition of the eye and should be used as the first step in photographing the anterior segment.

Optical Sectioning

The slit lamp derives its name from its ability to produce a fine thin beam, or "slit," of light that can be projected onto the cornea. Using this slit of light by itself, we can observe a cross-section of the different corneal layers (Figure 3.12). This thin slit beam is controlled by adjustments on the slit lamp illuminator. On the Zeiss photo slit lamp, these controls are located directly behind the slit beam housing; the two white levers control the height and width of the slit beam. When the lever closest to the slit beam housing is moved all the way to the left, a very fine thin beam appears. A metal stopper also located there can be set for three positions, from very

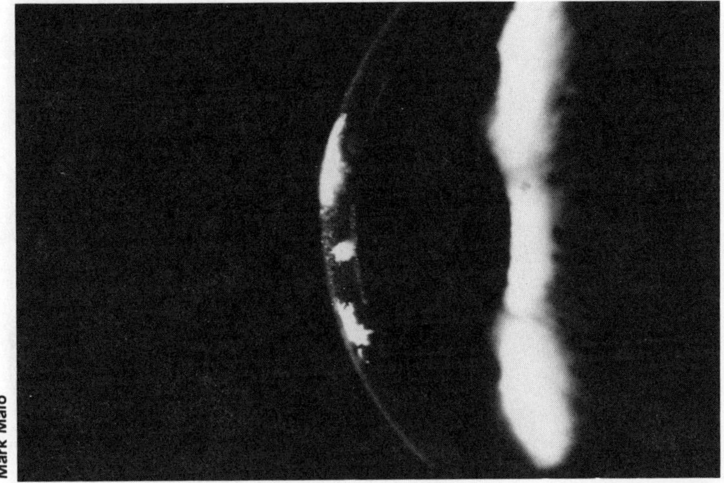

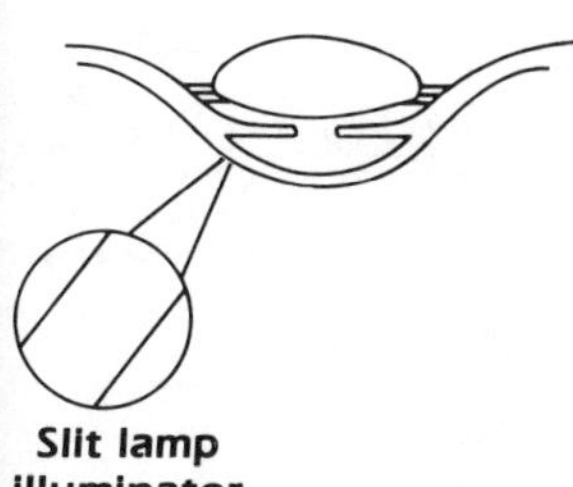

Figure 3.12 Optical section.

thin to moderately thin. Other photo slit lamps have variations of this control system.

The thin beam of light is best seen when the optical head is placed in at least a 30° angle to the slit lamp illuminator. An end-on view of the cornea is then observed, highlighting the epithelium, stromal, and endothelial layers so that a particular corneal disorder can be localized. A thin slit beam can also be used to reveal shape and elevation in certain corneal disorders. Also, comparing the thickness of different areas in the cornea of one eye, or of both eyes, is a primary use of the thin slit beam. Irregularities on the corneal surface show up very well when a thin slit beam is placed on the cornea.

A general rule for corneal slit lamp photography is to highlight surface irregularities by using a narrow beam with low diffuse background illumination. To highlight corneal infiltrates, edema, or opacities use a wider slit beam.

At times, recording elevation in the anterior segment presents a problem. The three-dimensional value through the oculars may fool the photographer into thinking that the lighting and view seen through the oculars will have the same dramatic effect on a single 35mm color slide. In order to avoid disappointment after reviewing the processed film, two rules must be remembered:

1. When trying to preview lighting as it will appear on film, close the eye that looks through the ocular without the reticule. If the view does not look as good, adjust the lighting to duplicate the effect viewed with both eyes open.
2. Choose a lighting technique that helps to accentuate the three dimensionality of the pathology.

Optical Section With Diffuse Illumination

This is probably the most useful and popular form of illumination in slit lamp photography. By projecting a thin slit

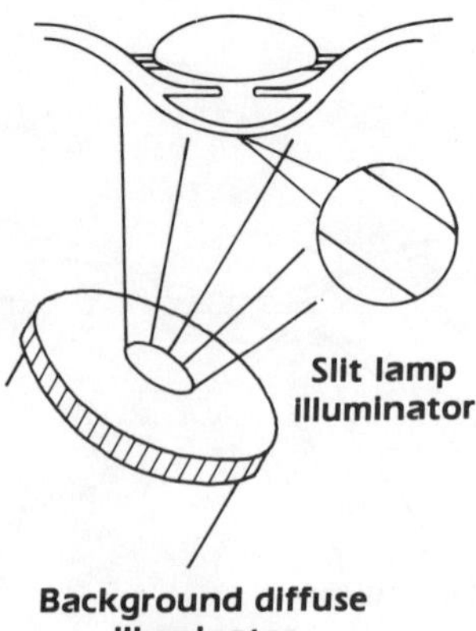

Figure 3.13 Optical section with diffuse illumination.

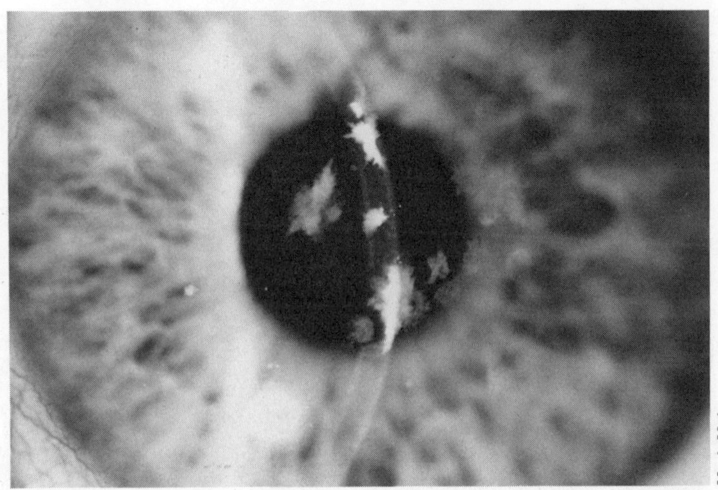

beam simultaneously with the diffuse-background illumination, one can obtain a general view of the eye and highlight a specific area of the cornea, especially corneal surface irregularities (Figure 3.13).

Broad Beam Illumination

Once the layer of depth of a pathologic condition has been established, the extent of corneal involvement needs to be recorded. This is accomplished with broad beam illumination (Figure 3.14). To achieve a broad beam, move the width-control lever on the slit beam illuminator to the right of center. The further to the right the lever is moved, the wider the beam will become. Moving the lever to the extreme right produces a full circle of light. Using a wide beam makes it easier to show fine corneal detail that otherwise might not show up in a thin optical section.

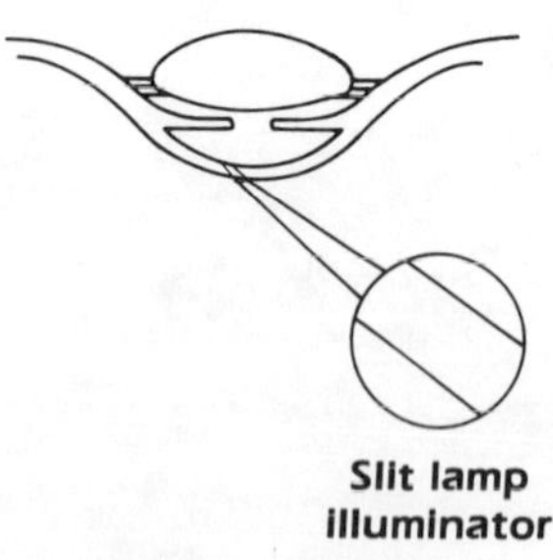

Figure 3.14 Broad beam illumination.

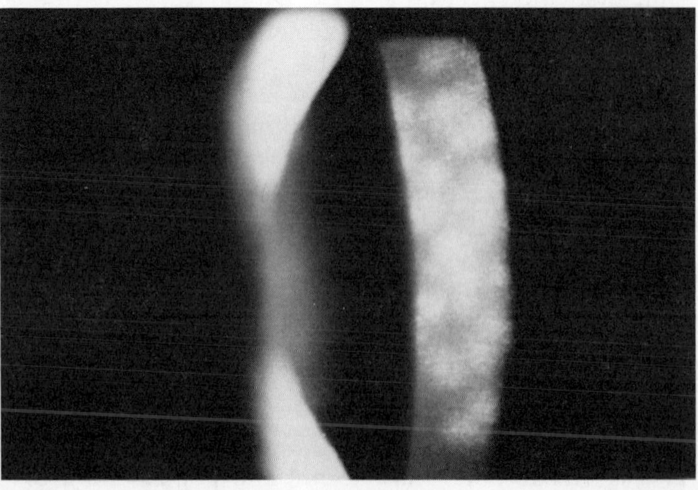

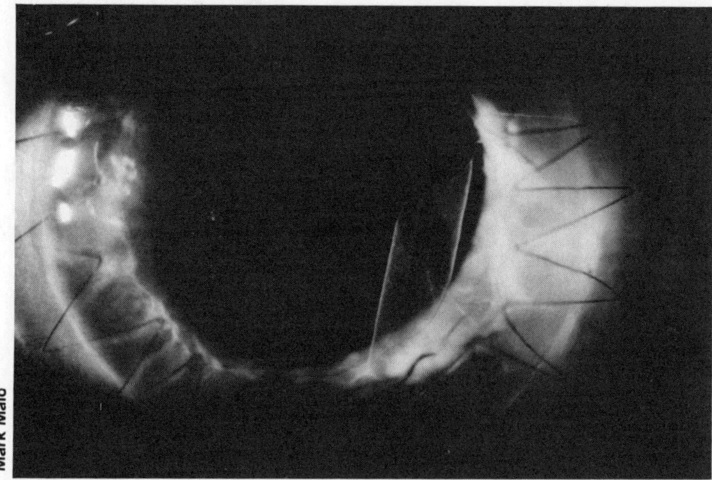

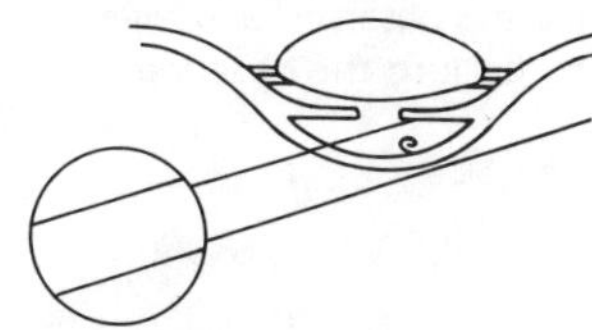

Figure 3.15 Tangential illumination.

Tangential illumination, by highlighting structures in the anterior segment with light directed from an extreme angle, helps show texture and dimension.

Tangential Illumination

When a broad light source is placed directly in front of the eye any pathology on the corneal surface will appear flat and without texture. Placing the light source to the extreme side of the subject produces shadows and enhances any texture (Figure 3.15). To best observe this effect, focus the slit lamp on a normal iris. Set the slit lamp illuminator for a wide circle, place the illuminator next to the optical head on the temporal side of the eye and focus the light on the iris. The diffuse background illuminator must be turned off to get the maximum effect of this lighting technique. While looking through the oculars, slowly move the light toward the temporal side of the eye. The further the light gets from the optical head, the more texture will be seen in the iris.

This technique can also be used to view pathology in the cornea or lens. To start, dilate the eye to be photographed. This will give a clear view of the lens, but more importantly, it will provide a dark background against which the pathology will be highlighted. In an undilated eye, light hitting the cornea will also hit the iris, causing the pathology to blend in with the iris. Using tangential illumination causes the light to fall across the pathology, lighting it up against the dark dilated pupil.

Indirect Illumination

In this section we will learn to take photography of the cornea one step further with the two most commonly used forms of indirect illumination, sclerotic scatter and retroillumination. Indirect illumination refers to the technique of illuminating pathological conditions not by the light that falls directly on it, but rather by light that strikes an adjacent area of the eye first. Bouncing the light off this area redirects it to the desired site from an angle not possible with direct illumination.

Retroillumination means light striking an object from a point behind both the object and the observer, and reflecting back to the observer.

Retroillumination is an indirect lighting technique that can be compared to producing a silhouette. When one views the sunset behind the skyline of a large city, one sees the tall buildings outlined by the bright light behind them. This same approach can be used in photographing pathological conditions in the anterior segment of the eye. Specifically, light can be reflected off the retina or the iris and the areas of pathologic interest located in front of them will appear in silhouette.

Retroillumination From the Fundus

The first step in retroillumination is dilation of the eye to be photographed so that light can be directed onto the retina without pupillary constriction. Light bouncing off the retina back toward the optical head of the photo slit lamp will silhouette any abnormalities in either the lens or the cornea (Figure 3.16). The colored pigment layer in the retina affects the color of the reflected light. Specifically, the retinas of Caucasian patients reflect an orange-red light, while those of Blacks, Hispanics, and Orientals tend to have a brown reflex.

In setting up the photo slit lamp for retroillumination, place the slit illuminator as close to the optical head as possible in a co-axial position. The light entering the eye from this position will bounce directly back through the lens of the eye and the cornea and any pathologic condition will be shown in silhouette.

When using this technique, make sure the shape of the slit beam entering the eye conforms to the opening through

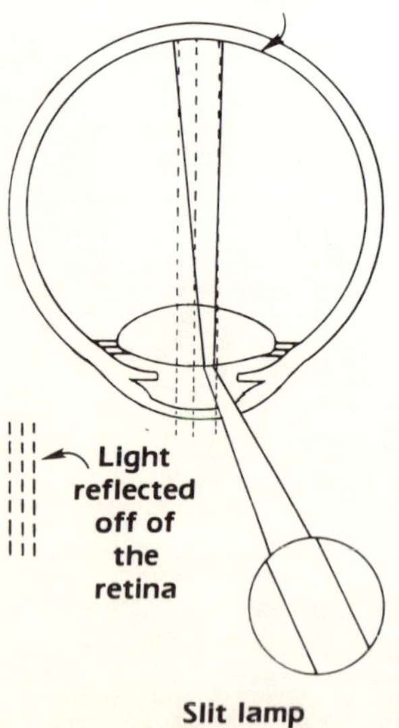

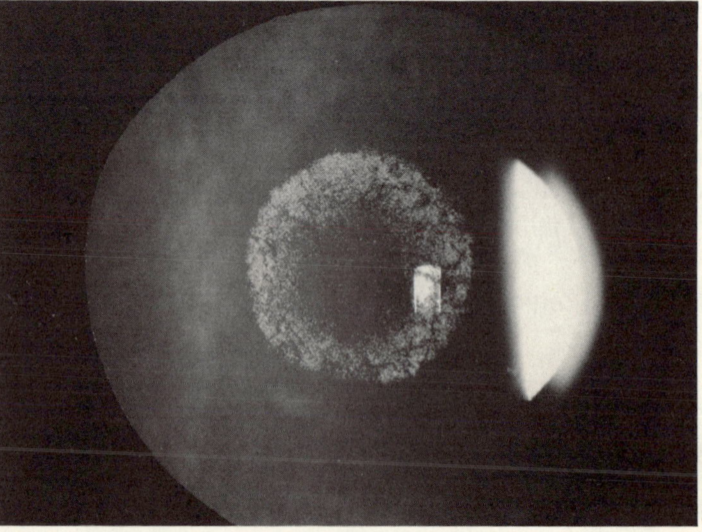

Figure 3.16 Retroillumination from the retina.

which it is being directed. For instance, adjusting the beam into a "crescent moon" shape will fit it nicely next to either edge of the iris. The crescent shape is made by placing the height adjustment lever on the slit lamp illuminator halfway between two of its settings. Care should be taken as to the size of this light; if the crescent is too big, light will hit the iris, which looks distracting in the final photograph. The darker pigmentation of some eyes prevents the reflection of an adequate amount of light back to the camera for a proper exposure. This problem may be overcome by having the patient shift his/her fixation to a position where the crescent strikes the optic nerve head. Light striking the optic nerve head will produce a bright yellow reflex, reflecting enough light for a proper exposure. The results of this technique can be quite dramatic, however, like most lighting techniques, retroillumination from the retina is most effective when used in conjunction with a series of photographs taken using other techniques.

Retroillumination From the Iris

Retroillumination from the iris is achieved by using the same lighting principles as that of retroillumination from the retina, except that the iris is not dilated (Figure 3.17). As a result, careful placement of the light source allows the photographer to observe corneal pathology by reflecting the slit beam of light off the iris, directly behind it. After adjusting the slit lamp illuminator to a tall, wide beam, focus on the corneal pathology. When the slit lamp illuminator is in its centered position, the broad beam will directly illuminate the pathology and help in achieving a critical focus. Without moving the focus, use the decentering control knob on the

Retroillumination is best achieved by using a slit beam equal in height to the surface the slit beam is to be passed through or reflected off. A 9mm slit beam will not fit into a 6mm pupil. The beam should not directly strike the surface being photographed.

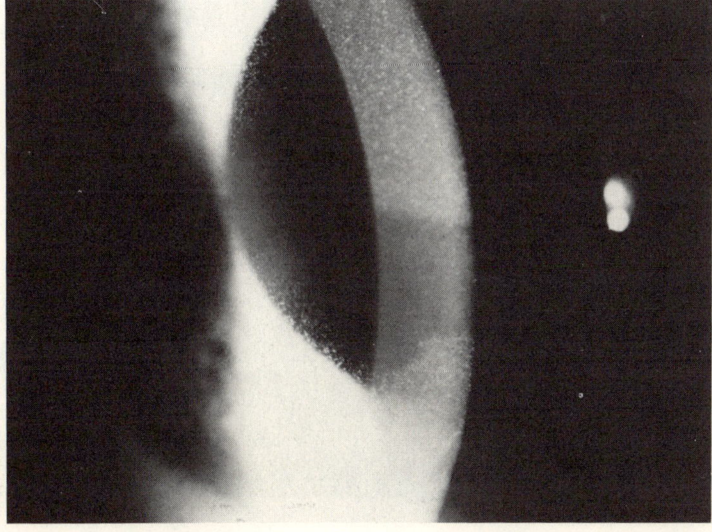

Mark Maio

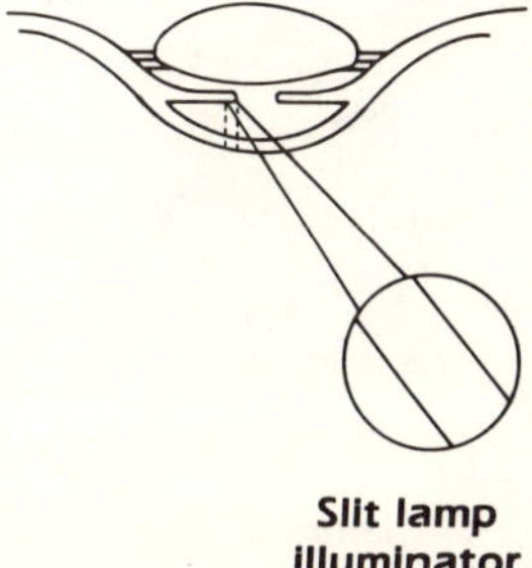

Figure 3.17 Retroillumination from the iris.

slit lamp illiminator to shift the beam of light to one side of the pathology. This slight movement will place the light beam on the iris directly behind the pathology and render it in silhouette. By varying this angle slightly, the photographer can observe subtle changes that add detail to the appearance of the pathology.

A secondary lighting technique can be created simultaneously with retroillumination from the iris. During iris retroillumination, a small dark zone exists between the area where the beam of light strikes the epithelial surface of the cornea and where it is reflected back off the iris. This indirect retroillumination from the iris may provide detail that is sometimes lost in direct retroillumination.

Sclerotic Scatter

Sclerotic scatter is an illumination technique whereby a slit beam of light is placed at the limbus and an internal light reflection is directed throughout the cornea, highlighting any abnormalities in the cornea.

Sclerotic scatter is a lighting technique used to highlight pathology that involves a majority of the cornea, rather than a small isolated area, as shown by other forms of illumination (Figure 3.18).

Setting up the photo-slit lamp for sclerotic scatter is similar to the initial steps of indirect retroillumination from the iris. With the diffuse illuminator turned off and the slit illuminator set in the centered position, place a tall, wide direct slit beam on the cornea. After focusing, decenter the beam and position it at the limbus (the junction of the cornea and the sclera); this will send light throughout the stromal layer of the cornea, allowing it to exit at the limbal areas which are not being directly illuminated by the slit beam. A ring of light will appear around the cornea when the light is correctly positioned, and any pathology will be highlighted by the light traveling through the cornea (Figure 3.18). No light reaches the iris in this procedure, and this provides a dark background for the illuminated corneal

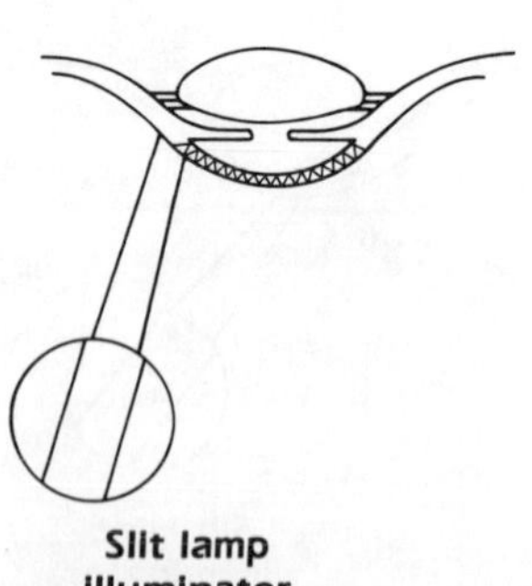

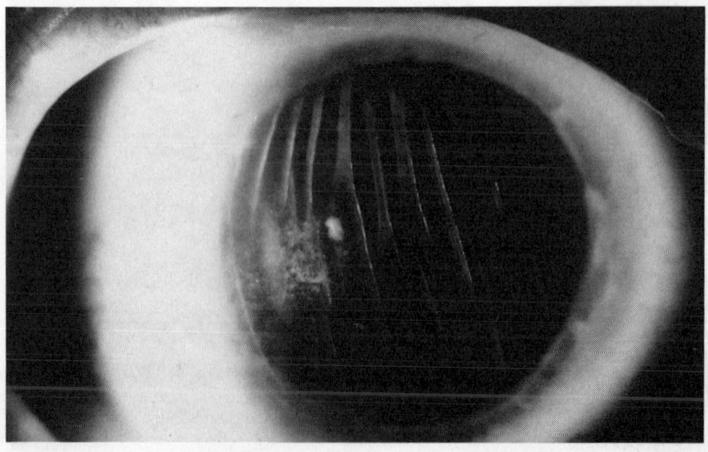

Figure 3.18 Sclerotic scatter.

pathology. This detailed view of the pathology can be indispensible in the photographic documentation of many corneal dystrophies.

One final illumination technique, Specular Reflection, will be treated in Chapter 4.

Using the Photo Slit Lamp

Establishing a System

As in any procedure, it is critical that a repeatable system be established prior to attempting photography. Mistakes are more easily corrected when one performs the mechanical steps of the photo slit lamp in a consistent manner and records the variations for each photograph in a notebook. Any unacceptable photographs compared with this information will quickly improve the photographer's technique.

The initial step of the photographer's system should be a photo slit lamp request form completely filled out by the physician with specific information regarding the type and location of pathology, and any suggested lighting techniques. This information should be recorded in a log book, and a nametag should be prepared. The nametag should be photographed with the photo-slit lamp before taking any clinical photos for easy patient photo identification. Finally, any adjustments to the room or camera should be made before bringing the patient in for photography.

Patient Management

Enough emphasis cannot be placed on the importance of patient management in ophthalmic photography. The ability of the photographer to manage the patient during the photographic session is as important as photographic technique. Regardless of the photographer's efforts, it is next to impossible to obtain quality photographs of an uninformed, uncomfortable patient. Photography should not be attempted until the photographer has spent as much time as necessary explaining the procedure and making any adjustments to the instrument.

A well-defined method for educating photographer and patient prior to beginning a photo session should be followed.

Alignment of the Photo Slit Lamp

Having the photo slit lamp in the proper position before the patient enters the room facilitates the photographic procedure and helps build patient confidence in the photographer; adjusting the photo slit lamp once the patient is in position may give the impression of uncertainty and inexperience.

The request sheet should be reviewed before the patient enters the photo room so that the photo slit-lamp can be set up and aligned for the proper eye. As for the actual set up, the slit lamp illuminator should be positioned on the temporal side of the eye to aid in providing a wide range of movements. Because the nasal side is limited by the extension of the nose, this technique also provides a landmark for establishing which eye has been photographed. When viewing the completed photograph and noting the origin of the slit beam the photographer can quickly identify the temporal side of the eye.

Magnification

Magnification on film is usually one power less than magnification in the slit lamp ocular. Pretest any new system.

Most photo slit lamps have a magnification range of 6x-25x, although some go as high as 40x (Figure 3.19).

Choosing which magnification to use for photography is closely related to the lighting technique selected. For instance, lighting techniques such as diffuse, optical section with diffuse, or sclerotic scatter are used to show the entire cornea. A 6x-16x magnification is required to permit this total view. Optical section, broad beam, tangential, and retroillumination are used to show more specific areas and tend to work best with magnifications in the 16x-40x range.

A common problem encountered when doing photography has to do with the fact that the camera "sees" an image one magnification lower than that viewed through the oculars (Figure 3.20). There are two ways of correcting this problem. The first can be applied to all slit lamps. View the eye at the desired final magnification and make all lighting adjustments. Just prior to making the exposure, increase the magnification to the next highest setting. The image recorded on the film will then match that of the first image

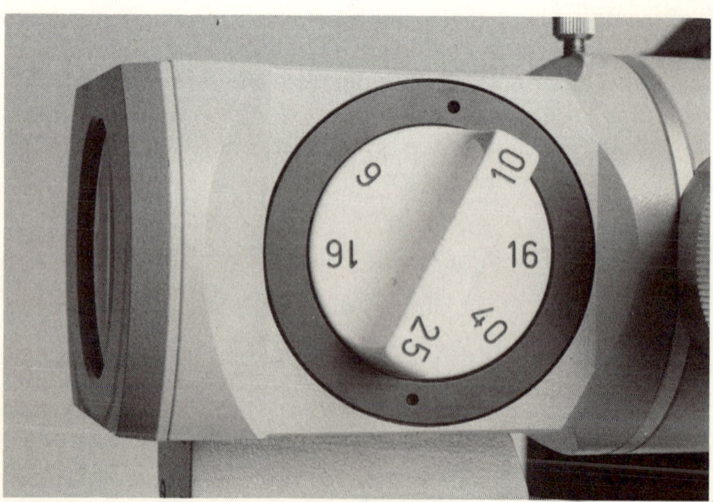

Figure 3.19 Magnification control wheel.

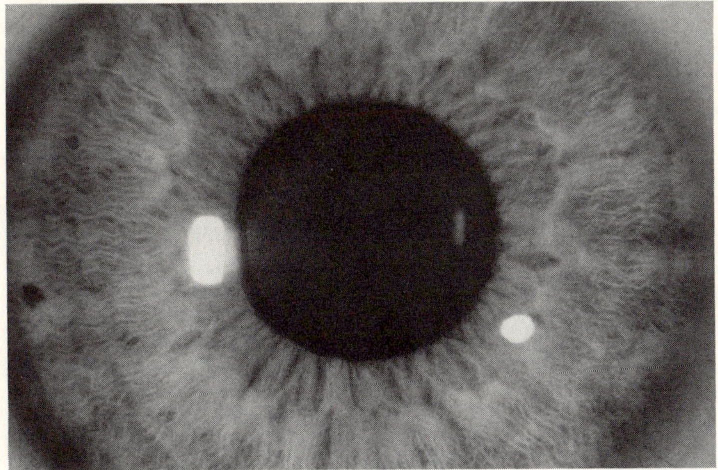

Figure 3.20 Photographer's view at 16x seen through the eyepieces.

viewed. The second solution involves installing a magnifier between the 35mm camera body and the optical head to magnify the image going to the camera to match that seen through the oculars. Thus, using one magnification for observation and another for photography is no longer necessary. Not all photo slit lamps allow this option, so one should check with the manufacturer.

Orientation of the 35mm Camera

Many photo slit lamps restrict the position of the 35mm camera to a horizontal format. While this is adequate for most photographs, there are times when a vertical position would be better suited to the subject. For example, when photographing a tall thin beam at 16x, a horizontal format will eliminate the top and bottom of the beam in the photograph (Figure 3.21). The entire slit beam of light may

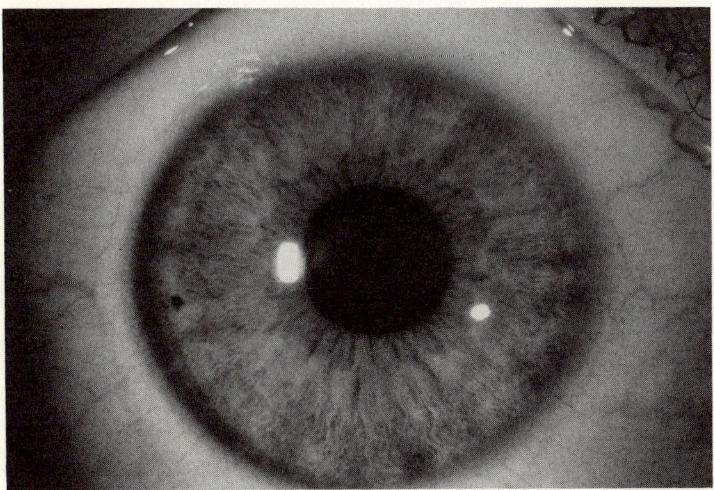

Figure 3.21 Magnification seen at the film plane when taking the photograph at 16x.

be recorded by rotating the 35mm camera to vertical position. While this option is not available on every photo slit lamp, using it on those cameras so equipped will help record as much information on one photograph as possible.

Film

An exposure test for each film used should be conducted prior to photographing patients.

Color slide film, which produces a color positive image and comes in a number of varieties and brands, is the standard for use in the photo slit lamp.

Film is classified according to its sensitivity to light; this is referred to as its ISO number. The higher this number is, the more sensitive to light that film is. Thus, a film with an ISO of 200 is twice as sensitive as one with an ISO of 100.

The type of film chosen depends greatly on the power source of the photo slit lamp because the latter vary greatly in the amount of light they generate. Those that generate a lower maximum output require color slide film in the 200-400 ISO range. Power sources with higher outputs allow use of film in the 64-200 ISO range.

Lower ISO films have a distinct advantage over the faster films in that they have the ability to render fine detail. Therefore, choosing the lowest possible ISO film that can be used on a given photo slit lamp assures the highest quality image possible.

Exposure

An understanding of how light affects film is needed before an intelligent decision can be made regarding the amount of light required to record a particular pathology, and the value of a basic photography class cannot be underemphasized. In addition, the large variety of films and photo-slit lamps available makes it impossible to formulate a definitive exposure guide for various pathologies. However, a "rule of thumb" can be given as a starting point. Lighter areas of pathology and structures of the eye reflect more light than darker areas. Thus, those areas reflecting more light will require less exposure to render a high quality image. Conversely, the darker the subject, the more light needed for proper exposure. Control of the amount of light is governed by f-stops in some cameras, and the selection of different power settings on others.

By applying this principle to an exposure test conducted with a specific photo slit lamp and film, an exposure guide can be developed for that particular combination. While doing the test, care should be taken to record all exposures in a log book. Variations such as magnification, type of illumination and power setting (or f-stop) should be noted. When the film is returned from being processed, these notations should be transferred to the cardboard slide mount. The photographs can be reviewed and the correct exposures noted. Further testing over a period of time will be required to fine tune this process.

A system should also be established for taking photographs. The "whole story" of the cornea's condition is best told with a series of photographs taken using different lighting techniques. These photographs act as building blocks, each adding information when viewed with the previous one. The complete series should answer any questions about the eye's condition. The most informative, ideal series might consist of a low magnification diffuse illumination photograph, an optical section with diffuse illumination and an optical section. Photographs taken with the other specific lighting techniques will add to this information.

Summary

The final challenge to becoming proficient in slit-lamp photography is pushing oneself past the point of accepting "success" as just the ability to record an image of the anterior segment on film. The photographer should constantly ask: "Is the photograph sharp enough? Is it taken with the appropriate magnification? Was the correct lighting technique used? Are there any distracting artifacts? Is this the best possible image?" The ultimate question should be, "Did I produce the photograph that was requested?" These questions can only be answered by constant review of the photographs, along with constructive criticism from the physician requesting them. Achieving a consistently high level of quality in photography comes with constant practice and patience.

CHAPTER 4

Specular Microscopic Photography

by Kirby Miller

In this chapter we will learn how to photograph the corneal endothelium with specialized cameras—specular microscopes.

The corneal endothelium is a single layer of hexagonally shaped cells on the posterior (back) surface of the cornea. The cornea and sclera comprise the outer coating of the eye. The cornea (Figure 4.1) is a five-layered transparent structure encompassing the front sixth of this ocular shell. The cornea acts as the main refracting (light bending) surface of the eye. Corneal endothelial cells act as a metabolic pump to balance the amount of water in the stroma (the middle layer) of the cornea to maintain its clarity. When corneal endothelial cells die they do not regenerate. The remaining cells swell in size and fill the space vacated by the dead cell. Instrumentation that allows a view of these cells gives ophthalmologists the opportunity to quantify the endothelium in terms of "cell count" common in many aspects of medicine and to make some qualitative judgments concerning the health and appearance of the cell structure.

The angle of incidence is equal to the angle of reflection. A rough irregular surface will scatter light at varying angles producing a diffusion of light rather than a bright reflection. A smooth mirror reflects incident light most completely at an equal and opposite angle.

This chapter will examine three instruments and their application to imaging and recording the appearance of the corneal endothelium: the clinical slit lamp/photo slit lamp; the noncontact specular microscope; the contact specular microscope. The clinical slit lamp can be used to evaluate successfully the corneal endothelium. The photo slit lamp modes add documentary capability to the clinical slit lamp. Both are noncontact. In the 1970s, with the addition of magnification, the contact specular microscope was introduced, and it offered significant advantages over the other two methods.

Slit Lamp

The clinical slit lamp (biomicroscope) was first used to describe the appearance of the five layers of the cornea as they appear in optic section. Vogt and others additionally describe seeing the

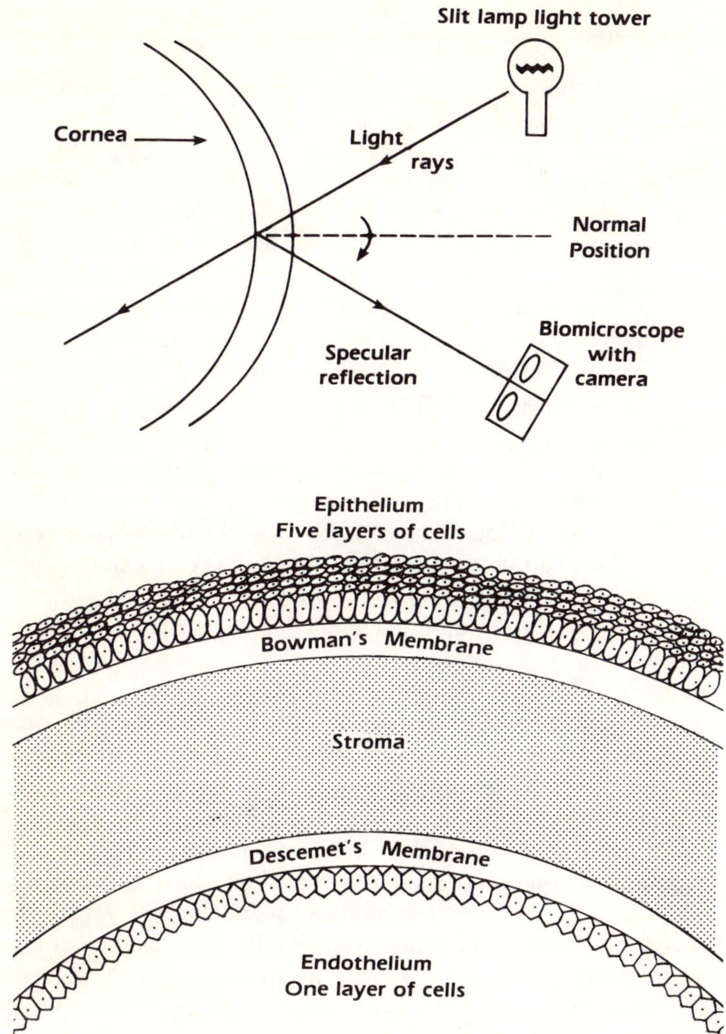

Figure 4.1 A schematic representation of the human cornea, with its five layers. Specular microscopy is usually done on the innermost layer of hexagonal cells, the endothelium.

individual endothelial cells using an illumination technique called specular reflection. A specular reflection is a bright "mirror like" reflex observed when the angle of incidence of the light source and the angle of reflection to the observer are equal. This is commonly seen in daily experience. When bright highlights are seen dancing on the surface of a lake, one is observing specular reflection with the angle of the sunlight and the observer's position being equal. This same phenomenon can be used to advantage with the slit lamp, as the cornea is a smooth evenly curved reflecting surface. Although the ability to manipulate the slit lamp to image the endothelium is documented in ophthalmic literature, it was rediscovered following the introduction of contact specular microscopes in the 1970s.

Technique

There are three concepts to keep in mind when learning to use the slit lamp to image the endothelium:

1. The angle of the slit beam and the position of the observer, coincident with the optic head of the slit lamp, must be equal and opposite, that is, with the patient gazing straight ahead the slit beam is 30 ° to the right side, the optical head 30° to the left of the axis of fixation (Figure 4.2).
2. This technique is essentially monocular. The cells will appear much better in one ocular (eyepiece) of the slit lamp.
3. Magnification is extremely important. When many clinicians speak of seeing the endothelium, they are observing the general appearance of the corneal endothelial mosaic rather than visualizing individual cells. Using the highest available magnification or adding a specular magnifying eyepiece will greatly facilitate this technique.

A good representation of cells seen with the slit lamp is shown in Figure 4.2. This photograph, taken with a Zeiss photoslit lamp, shows large cells with dark areas. These areas are corneal guttata. Conditions in which large cells are present are more easily seen than those with normal cells. Additionally, cell estimates are easier when there are fewer cells to count.

Specular reflexes from the corneal epithelium are common during slit lamp examination. When specular reflexes are seen, they are generally ignored. To see the endothelium, the first step is simply to place the slit beam tower at 30° from the central axis of forward fixation, and sweep the cornea until a bright specular reflex is seen. This will happen because at some point the angle of incidence will equal the angle of reflection. This first step should be performed at low magnification, especially for those uncomfortable with the shallow focus at higher magnifications or who may be unfamiliar with the slit lamp.

When the bright reflex is seen, the cells can be observed immediately adjacent to this reflex. By increasing the magnification and focusing slightly more posterior to the cornea, the cells will be seen in the dark field adjacent to the area where the bright reflex was seen (Figure 4.2). For example, if one is examining a left eye with the slit beam at 30° and positioned temporally, the field of cells will be seen to the left of the bright reflex.

Fortunately, it is much more difficult to describe this technique than it is to actually perform it. Some practice and experimentation on the part of the examiner is necessary. The important consideration is to first achieve a view of recognizable cells. As with all methods of endothelial imaging, only a very small percentage of light for observation will return to illuminate the cells; the low contrast of the cells

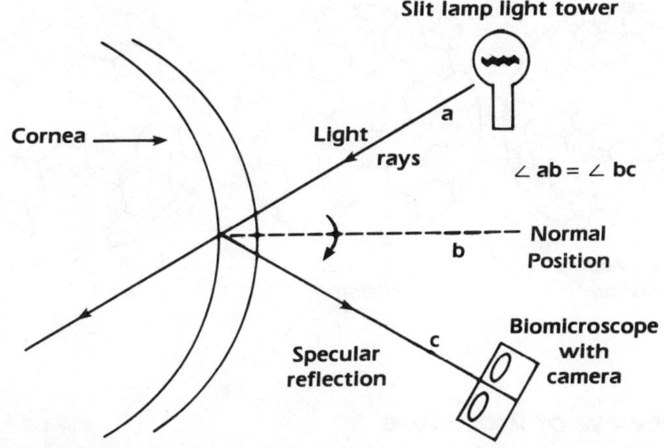

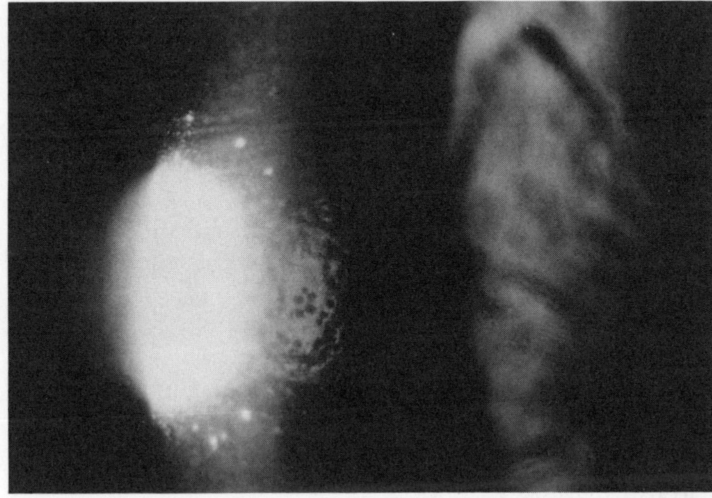

Figure 4.2 Illumination techniques for slit lamp specular microscopy. An example of this technique. Note the tiny endothelial cells immediately to the right of the bright reflex.

also makes this more difficult. Two refinements will become apparent after some experience. It is helpful to reduce the height of the slit beam after the specular reflex has been achieved. This will reduce some useless light scatter and glare. Additionally, it will be observed that there is a compromise involving the width of the slit. A relatively thin slit should be used initially. This yields the greatest contrast and definition of the cell borders. As the slit width is increased a greater field of cells is observed, but the increased light scatter tends to decrease the contrast. There will be a zone where the widest field of cells can be seen with the greatest definition. This will vary depending on the thickness of the corneas and the presence of any changes anterior to the endothelium that may scatter additional light.

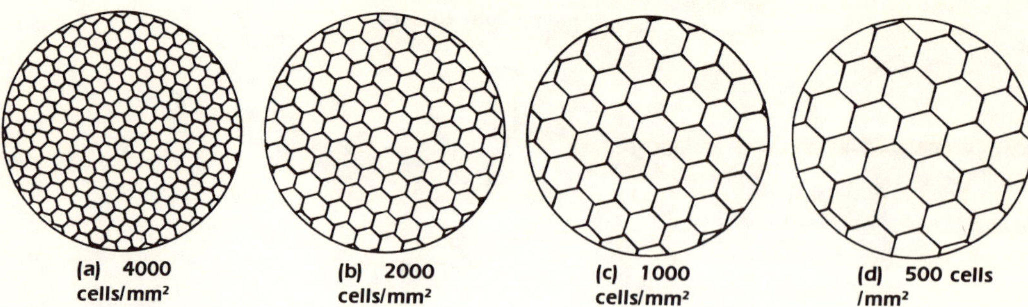

Figure 4.3 Representation of various cell populations: (a) $4000/mm^2$ (b) $2000/mm^2$ (c) $1000/mm^2$ (d) $500/mm^2$. Appearance varies with the model of slit lamp being used.

Review of Procedure

Instrumentation

A biomicroscope with magnification of 25x or above is suitable. Inserts for additional magnification which are slipped into the tube are available for other slit lamps.

Technique

1. Start with a moderately thin slit at 30°.
2. Sweep the cornea looking for a bright reflex from the epithelium.
3. Increase the magnification and carefully focus the endothelial cells.
4. Adjust the slit width and height for maximum field and definition.

Quantification

The Mosaic Matcher was developed by Dr. John Karickhoff of Falls Church, Virginia. It has been calibrated for several slit lamps and may be available through the slit lamp manufacturer or by contacting Dr. Karickhoff.

The counting of cells with the slit lamp is an estimate, as are all methods. The Mosaic Matcher is a helpful tool (Figure 4.3). Dr. Holladay and others suggest a method based on the projection of the slit as a fixed field. The eyepiece attachments have grids to facilitate counting the cells.

It is strongly recommended that the technician not operate in a void when performing endothelial cell counts. If the slit lamp method can be mastered with confidence and all that is desired is a cell count, then the more expensive instruments are not necessary. Photography of the cells is only possible with a photo slit lamp, however, so hard copy documentation is often impossible. For those who are using the noncontact or contact specular microscopes, use of the slit lamp can be very important to identify zones where a view of the endothelium can be achieved in compromised corneas and to check for any conditions that may make con-

Dr. Holladays's method is presented in "Quantitative Endothelial Biomicroscopy," **Journal of Ophthalmic Surgery,** January, 1983.

tact specular micrography more difficult. In addition, mastery of cell counting using the slit lamp provides a back up to an existing specular micrography system.

Noncontact Specular Microscopy

The broadest definition of noncontact specular microscopy would certainly include the biomicroscope. The development of specific instruments designated by this term, however, came much later. Following the introduction of contact specular microscopes and accompanying revelations in endothelial research, many clinicans desired a method to view and photograph the endothelium, but could not justify the expense and dedication of a single instrument for such a specialized purpose. As a result, noncontact microscopes were developed.

For many years, Nikon produced a noncontact specular microscope that also performed high magnification slit image photography (Figure 4.4). Unfortunately this instrument is no longer being marketed. The remaining noncontact systems are provided by Carl Zeiss, Inc. and Topcon Corporation.

It is important to note that these instruments are attachments for existing slit lamps, either clinical examination units or photo slit lamps. Basically, these instruments offer increased magnification to the existing instrument. For this reason, their operation is similar to the previous discussion of the use of the slit lamp to illuminate the endothelial cell layer.

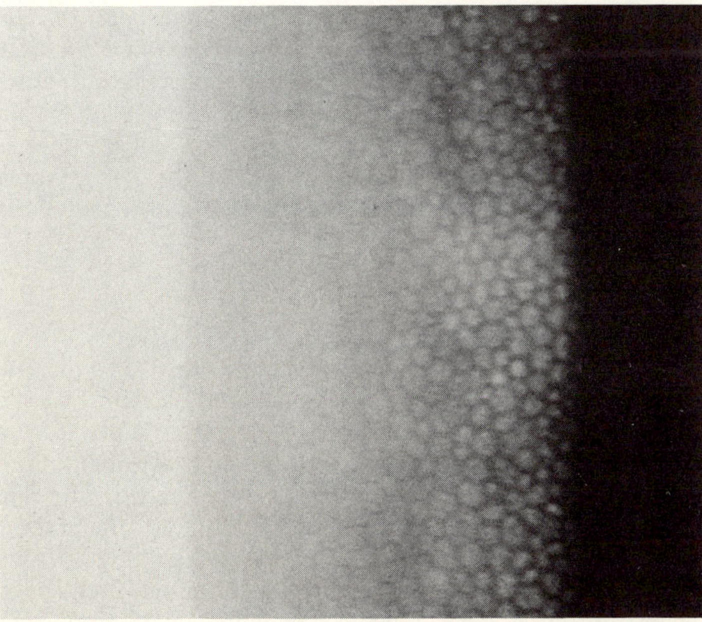

Figure 4.4 A field of cells taken with a Zeiss noncontact specular microscope. The right reflex is decentered and illuminates the strip of cells. The cells are obviously more easily seen than with the lower magnification slit lamp seen in Figure 4.2.

Procedure

Instrumentation

It is necessary to remove the front objective lens from the slit lamp. The noncontact attachment is placed in that position.

Technique

Use of the slit lamp for endothelial cell counts is limited by the magnification of the instrument relative to cell size. User unfamiliarity with the use of the slit lamp can make use of the non-contact microscope difficult to master.

1. Keeping the slit lamp technique in mind, the slit is placed at 30° and the cornea is swept with a moderately wide slit until a broad bright band is visualized. This is the specular reflex.
2. The instrument is then focused posterior on the cornea until a band of cells comes into view. The bright reflex will decenter in the field of view.
3. Total magnification will be a function of the selector on the slit lamp.
4. Once again, field size and cell definition can be manipulated by broadening the slit width.

Position the slit beam on the patient's cornea, while observing from the side of the slit lamp before moving to the oculars to observe the cells.

The magnification added by noncontact endothelial attachment introduces some difficulty for those disturbed by high magnification. It is often helpful, when learning to look at the patient's cornea with unaided vision to focus the slit image there before looking through the oculars of the biomicroscope. With such high magnification, small movements of the slit lamp joy stick introduce problems. The technician will quite often see elongated cells of the epithelium and artifacts of the stroma as the scope is focused. Shifting to lower magnification is not particularly helpful because of the vignetting or masking at the end of the attachments. For this reason, if the examiner is not seeing cells and is unsure of the position of the slit on the eye, he must look at the eye away from the instrument and recenter the slit beam.

Quantification

The noncontact attachments use a fixed field system. The cells may be estimated when viewed on a clinical microscope or from photographs when attached to a photo slit lamp.As a general rule, five separate fields of the central endothelium should be photographed and the results averaged. The film used for endothelial photography with these attachments should be of relatively high sensitivity, such as 400 ISO. The most common film is black and white, although high speed color transparency film may be used when a darkroom is not available. Cells may be counted directly from black-and-white negatives using hand held magnifiers, projected onto a screen with an overlay grid, or enlarged onto photographic paper. Each print or projected image should be of the same standard size so cell density calculations are uniform and comparable.

These cell counting aids offer significant advantage over the use of the biomicroscope by itself. The additional magnification makes cell counting easier and increases visibility of intracellular detail.

Contact Specular Microscopy

The contact microscope fostered the modern interest in the corneal endothelium. It was developed following the publication of an article by Dr. David Maurice in 1968 in which he described a technique for examining and photographing excised corneal endothelium. To do this Dr. Maurice created an instrument that was able to separate the illuminating light from that reflected back to the observer and see the corneal endothelium. Dr. Maurice viewed the endothelium at magnifications as high as 400x. This technique was quite a departure from the low magnifications of the clinical slit lamp and fostered the development of commercially available microscopes. Although the early instruments were somewhat difficult to use, current technology has solved many problems and made the instrument common outside the research laboratory.

Presently, there are contact microscopes available from CooperVision, Keeler, and BioOptics. These instruments have some differences, but their operation is similar enough to allow generalization about their operation (Figure 4.5).

The primary feature of these instruments is the microscope housing or optical head. The internal optics of these microscopes project a beam of light on one near normal axis onto the cornea and return the reflected light on a separate axis for observation and recording. As with the slit lamp technique, this angle of incidence of illuminating light is equal to the angle of reflection of observed light. More than 99 of the incident light pases through the cornea into the aqueous. Less than 1% is reflected back to the observer.

The field of view produced is determined by the maginfication available from the specific optical system in use. Applanation cones may be changed to increase or decrease the magnification and field of view. The early contact microscopes produced a narrow slit-like field of view at 200x magnification. Several researchers and clinicans wanted to see more of the endothelium in a single frame. This led to the development of "wide field" microscopes. In simple terms less magnification yields a wider field of view. One need only

Wide field microscopes offer qualitative and quantitative advantages to the user. Qualitative advantages are: brightness and contrast of image, easier evaluation, better appreciation of cell size variety, relocation of the same area is easier. Quantitative advantages are: more cells/picture, more accurate cell counts, and fewer pictures taken.

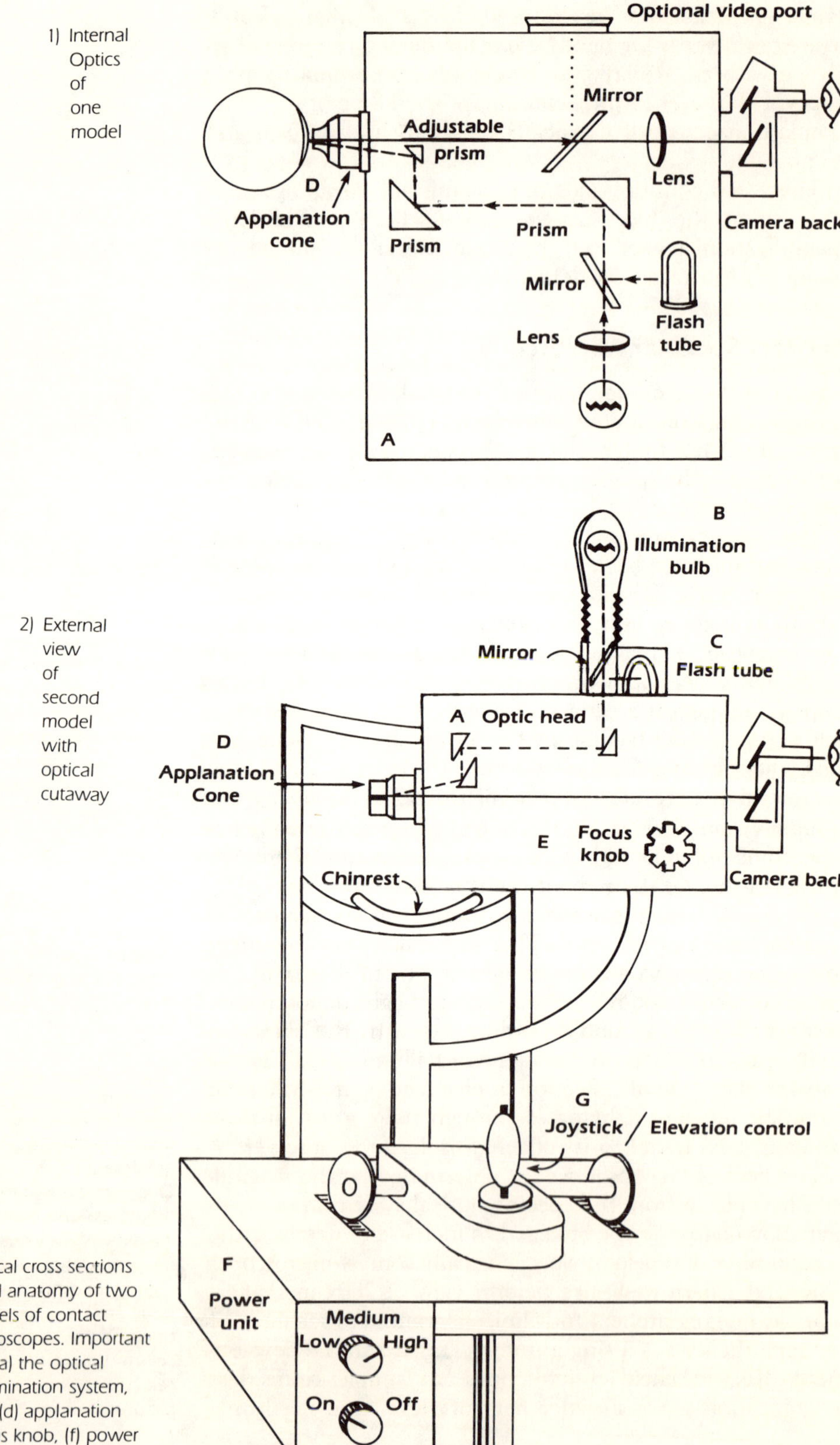

Fig. 4.5 Optical cross sections of the internal anatomy of two different models of contact specular microscopes. Important features are: (a) the optical head, (b) illumination system, (c) flash unit, (d) applanation cone, (e) focus knob, (f) power unit, (g) joystick control lever.

recall the discussion of the compromise between contrast and field with the slit lamp technique of specular microscopy to gain insight into the problems inherent in producing a wide field of cells with good definition.

The optical head is essentially a horizontal monocular microscope. There is an illumination source that projects light through the applanation cone and onto the cornea through a series of prisms. Most modern systems do not allow easy access to the adjustments for these prisms. It is necessary, however, for these prisms to be adjusted to produce the brightest, most efficient light exiting the microscope at the objective lens (the applanation cone in the contact mode). Microscopes can lose calibration and require recalibration by product representatives. If the particular system is designed to produce a video image, the light produced by the illumination housing is all that is required. If the system is designed to produce an image on film, there will be a flash tube assembly inserted in the illumination housing.

The light produced by the illumination housing is projected from the microscope at the objective lens and into the applanation cone. The cone is applanated onto the patient's cornea in a manner similar to applanation tonometry. The possibility of damaging the cornea is remote. Technicians who routinely perform applanation tonometry or A-Scan echography should be very comfortable with this procedure. This is one area where the available instruments differ to some degree. The Keeler scope has a fixed resistance function that signals an audible tone when unnecessary pressure is being exerted on the cornea. The CooperVision instrument has a traditional spring resistance cone. Both of these flatten the cornea to some degree to produce a solid applanation and a flat field of cells to view and photograph. The BioOptics features a concave applanation cone designed to ride on the tear film with minimal compression of the cornea. Instrument manuals correctly emphasize the strict necessity of keeping the applanation cones clean. Debris from the tear film can collect during the course of examination and produce artifacts on the final image. These may be seen as areas of fuzzy "clouds" on some instruments or small half circles on others. Some patients with oily tear film or eye makeup floating in the tear film may necessitate cleaning the lens before the second eye is applanated.

The optic head also contains a method for focusing the cells. This may be a knob or, in the case the Keeler instrument, motor driven focus operated within the joystick. It is important to know that these scopes can be prefocused at the approximate depth of the endothelium. The normal cornea is approximately .55 mm thick in the center. If the microscope has a pachymeter attached, it can be dialed in at about

The normal corneal thickness central is 0.49 to 0.56mm. The cornea thickness peripherally ranges from 0.70 to 0.90mm. Obviously, focus must be adjusted if counts are to be obtained close to the corneal limbus. These areas may be of particular interest, especially in postoperative patients. Since cataract incisions are peripheral, cells in those areas spread and migrate to cover cells compromised by the trauma of surgery. There may be disparity between central and peripheral cell counts in this group of patients.

The choice of using video as opposed to photographic methods to record cell counts is best determined by end use of such counts. Any time publication or use for teaching is required, still photography is the best choice for image clarity and resolution.

.45mm before the cornea is applantated. The Keeler scope has an indication of the thickness of the cornea viewed through a simple gauge at the top of the optic head. It is more efficient to prefocus the microscope, applanate the cornea and then fine focus the endothelial cells. This will greatly facilitate the examination and minimize the applanation time.

The image of the focused cells exits the microscope and is recorded in one of two methods. The CooperVision and Keeler microscopes both offer video systems. The cells are viewed on a video monitor with a video cassette recorder (VCR) in operation. The cornea is applanated, the VCR engaged in the record mode, and the cells focused. The best field is selected on playback, the recorder placed in pause, and the field photographed on Polaroid print film for a hard copy. Thirty-five millimeter cameras are also available for the Keeler. The Bio-Optics scope uses 35mm format exclusively. Generally, cells are photographed on black and white film of high sensitivity (ISO). Conventional negative films have the disadvantage of requiring processing before counts can be made. The newer Autoprocess Polaroid transparency black and white films offer quick in-house processing and are widely used for this purpose.

The selection of video versus 35mm has become a real problem for many technicians. Video offers an almost instant cell count. However, the resolution of current monitors, especially when the video tape recorder is placed in a pause mode is severely limited and image quality is greatly compromised. Conventional black and white films offer the highest degree of resolution and hence the best quality when reproduced in a positive print. In a situation where publication quality prints of endothelial photographs are required, 35mm is the primary choice. Keeler and CooperVision have recently attempted to deal with this dilemma by offering simultaneous video and 35mm. These instruments are not yet widely in use.

The base of the instruments has several features for gross positioning of the applanation cone. Beneath the patient chin rest, there is a cross slide to put the applanation cone in front of the correct eye. The joy stick is also used in positioning but should not be used when applanating the cornea. There is a fine adjustment knob which controls all movement toward the cornea. An additional elevation mechanism raises and lowers the applanation cone.

Technique

1. Screen the patient. It is strongly suggested that the person doing the specular microscopy examine the patient with the slit lamp prior to the procedure.

Listed here is a step-by-step guide to contact specular microscopy. Overcoming the fear of touching the patient's eye with the cone is the greatest barrier to mastering this photographic technique.

The ordering physician may not be familiar with some of the limitations of the technique. Look for dry eyes. The combination of a compromised tear film and a dry applanation cone can result in epithelial defects. Keep the cone wet with a non-saline tears solution. Look for pathology. Does the patient have a thickened cornea? This will require a significant change in level of focus and may prevent imaging the cells at all. Is the cornea clear? An important limitation of specular microscopy is that more advanced corneal problems prevent a view of the endothelium. Look for the obvious, such as contact lenses or intraocular lenses.

2. Check the microscope. The whole system should be operational before the eye is touched. Check the VCR or load the film. At this point the technician can prefocus the microscope by whatever method is available. Clean the applanation cone. Alcohol can be used together with a soft swab.
3. This procedure is impossible in the face of poor patient cooperation. One should use whatever persuasive techniques necessary to assure patients that this is important and they need to help. A professional attitude helps. Patients need to know to fixate carefully, keep chin and forehead in contact with the head rest and breathe in a relaxed manner. The technician may want to fire a few demonstration frames if using a 35mm camera back. Arrange equipment carefully so that the video monitor does not become an obtrusive fixation device for the patient.
4. Anesthesize the cornea with a topical anesthetic such as ophthaine.
5. Wet the applanation cone. Remember to watch for artifacts caused by tear film during the course of the examination.
6. Position the patient, reemphasizing the need for maximum cooperation. Turn the room lights off or very low. Remember that only a small fraction of the available light is used to image a surface with minimal contrast. A red light bulb or the light from a video monitor is sufficient to guide movements during the procedure.
7. Get into position. At this point the technician should be at the side of the camera so that he can view the end of the applanation cone and the cornea. Do not move behind the camera where the cornea is out of view. There will be time to shift to that position when necessary. At times, the technician's position may cause the patient to look at him rather than the fixation device.

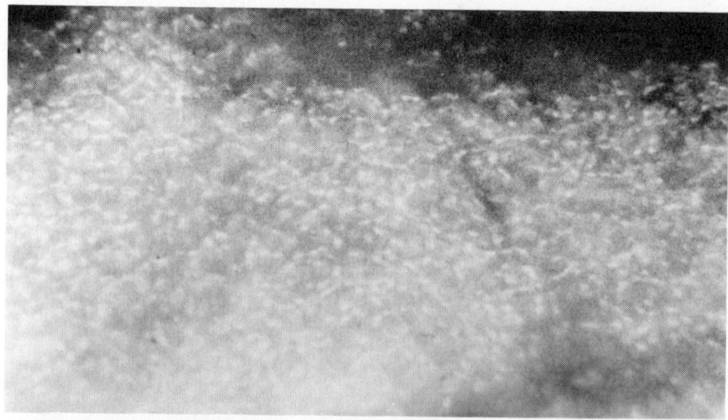

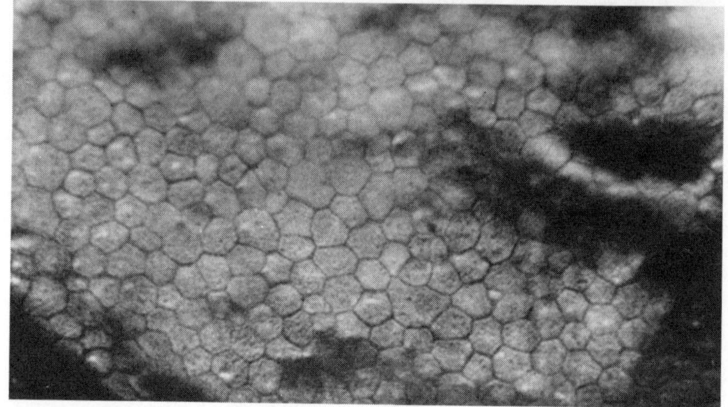

Figure 4.6 Wide field views of the corneal epithelium (top) and corneal endothelium (bottom).

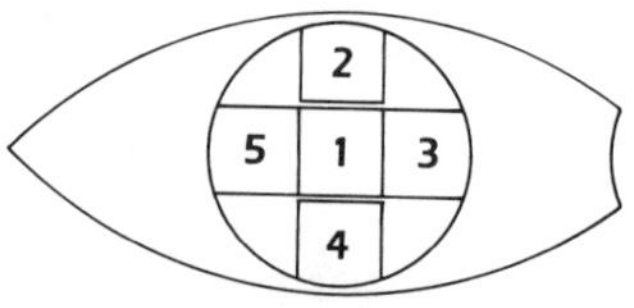

Five separate wide fields to cover central and peripheral cornea.

Figure 4.7 A photo plan to document various areas of the same cornea. Applanate within the five fields outlined by the solid lines. Such a pattern allows repetition and comparison. The fields do not overlap.

Patients should be cautioned against doing this before the cornea is applanated.

8. Bring the scope into gross position in front of the eye using the cross slide, joy stick, and elevation mechanism. As the cornea is approached, make small movements and aim for an area just slightly inferior to the apex of the cornea.
9. Applanate the cornea. Look for a bright reflex as the cone touches the tear film. It will be obvious that the light from the cone is scattering at the epithelial surface (Figure 4.6). The refraction of the light will pass onto the tear film. This indicates that the technician is close to a correct, flat applanation. Only a small additional movement of the positioning knob toward the cornea should be necessary.
10. Focus the cells (Figure 4.6.). At this point, attention should be directed toward either the video monitor or the camera eyepiece. If the scope has been correctly prefocused, the cells should be seen quickly.
11. Record the image or document on film. Again, five fields should be applanated and recorded for the count; one centrally and four in the quadrants around the central area (Figure 4.7). Although some

examiners move the cone while applanated, this is inadvisable, especially for the first 25 patients.

12. Examine the patient with the slit lamp and then congratulate him for his cooperation. If there is any question of corneal abrasion, he should be sent back to the clinic for examination by the referring ophthalmologist. If you are uncomfortable with releasing the patient, use this opportunity to look at the patient with the doctor and learn some slit lamp technique.

Quantification

The final step in performing specular micrography is to perform a cell count. Refer to the instructions provided for the instrument being used to properly determine the manner to count number of cells within the area photographed. Multiply this cell count as instructed in your camera manual to arrive at a final cell count.

Magnification varies with each system used, and with different applanation cones for the same contact systems. Double check the cell multiplying factor to insure a correct count. Cross check cell counts against a normal count to periodically check accuracy and microscope calibration.

Pitfalls in Technique

Uneven applanation can cause distortion of the view of the endothelium. If the end of the applanation cone is not making even contact with the corneal surface, the cells will appear to have a three dimensional appearance. Incomplete or uneven applanation will also prevent focusing the entire fields of cells, especially noticeable on the wide field instruments.

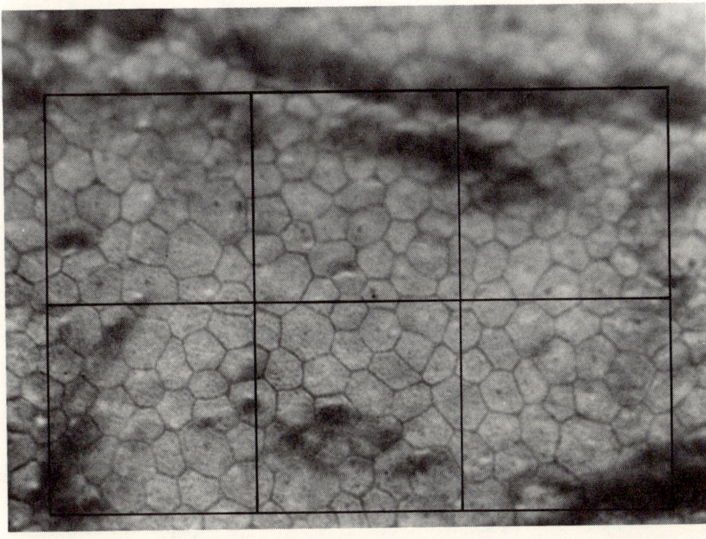

Figure 4.8 Cell counting with a grid. Count all complete cells contained within the grid lines as well as those touching one vertical and one horizontal axis. Surface irregularities prevent even focus.

All steps that can be accomplished prior to actually contacting the patient's cornea should be done prior to bringing the patient up to the chinrest.

Keeping the cone clean will prevent significant problems. It should be cleaned both prior to and following each examination. Dried salt crystals from saline solutions can scratch the cone as well as the patient's cornea. The cone should always be wet before it is touched with a swab. Although some examiners use a viscous gonio gel solution to facilitate moving the cone while on the eye, this causes more problems than it solves by gumming up the interface between the cone and the epithelial surface.

Count cells from more than one area to ensure accurate counts. Remember cell populations can vary in different locations on the same cornea.

Rapid, small eye movements are always present during the procedure. Unfortunately, the cataract population may also suffer from other medical conditions that cause additional movement it is helpful to have these patients control their breathing much in the same way as the radiologists when performing X-ray. Ask the patient to take a breath and hold it. You should applanate, focus, and record. This requires quick action by the technician and certainly can be challenging.

Tips: Keep the cone clean. Ask the patient to hold his breath during photography. Use a plano contact lens for children.

Children are also challenging subjects for this technique; they are best done by *noncontact* systems. It can be helpful to place a plano, high water contact lens on their eyes and tell them that this will protect the eye. Depending on the age of the child, this may be highly persuasive. Soft lenses can be used on any eye that is compromised for some reason, but this has not been found to be routinely necessary.

Summary

Examination of the corneal endothelium may be accomplished using the clinical slit lamp, noncontact specular microscope attachments, or the specialized contact specular microscope. Each method provides a quantitative evaluation of the health of the cornea by the ophthalmologist.

CHAPTER 5

Retinal Fundus Photography

by J. Michael Coppinger

The Retinal Fundus Camera

In this chapter we will learn how to perform retinal fundus photography. We will start with the special type of camera designed to photograph the inside of the eye, specifically the back lining of the eye, the retina. The three principal parts of a fundus camera (identical to those in a conventional camera) are an imaging system (optics), a recording mode (exposure by light), and a permanent means of image storage (film). The recording of the image of the retina is useful to the ophthalmologist for documenting and diagnosing pathology (Figure 5.1).

The principles of the indirect ophthalmoscope and the fundus camera work in the same manner with the same intent, that is, to put the observer's pupil within the patient's pupil to see into the back of the patient's eye. The indirect lens and the fundus camera place the photographer on the rim of a large hollow cave looking in. The camera is the eye we use to "see the sights" within.

A fundus camera combines the optical properties of a conventional camera with those of an indirect ophthalmoscope (Figure 5.2). An indirect ophthalmoscope uses a special aspheric lens to focus light into a patient's eye, then gathers the reflected light at a point in space between the lens and the observer's eyes. This real aerial image is inverted and backward. The observer/user views this image with a headset equipped with lenses, somewhat like a pair of glasses. A fundus camera uses this indirect lens system to form a real aerial image within a telescopic tube. The indirect lens is mounted on the front of the tube, a camera at the other end.

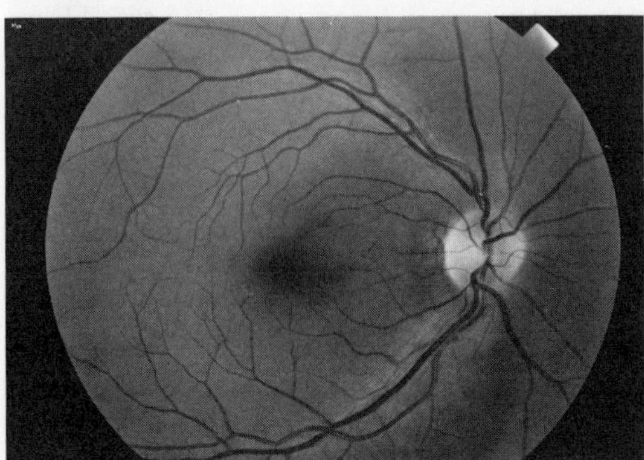
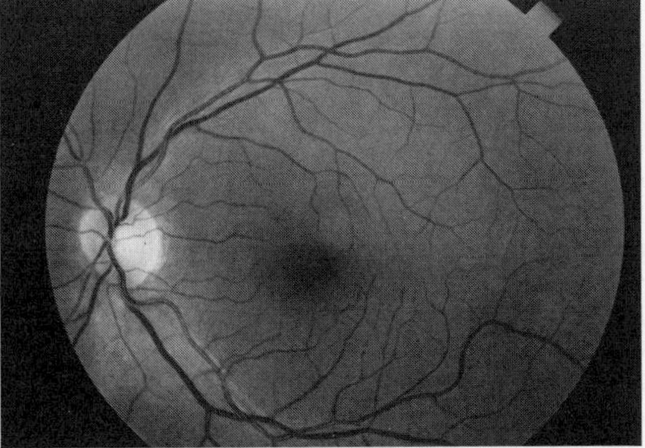

Figure 5.1 Fundus photos of the right eye (OD) and left eye (OS) of the same patient. The patient's nose lies between the two pictures. Optic disks, from which retinal arteries and veins enter and exit the sensory retina are located "nasal" to the dark central spot of sharpest visual acuity, the fovea of each eye.

Indirect Ophthalmoscope Simplified

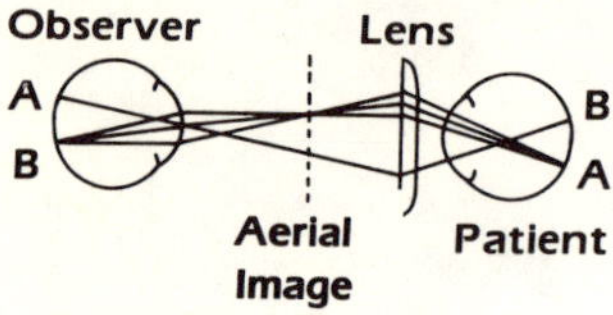

Figure 5.2 A simplified version of the principle of indirect ophthalmoscopy. The lens creates an image in space of the patient's retina that the observer views.

A second set of lenses within the tube reverts this image onto the film plane of a 35mm (or other type) of camera (Figure 5.3). The addition of an illumination/exposure system to this telescope permits photography. Fundus photography is the photographing of an aerial image produced by an indirect ophthalmoscope.

Retinal fundus cameras are either mydriatic (requiring patients to be dilated) or nonmydriatic (no dilation required). This section treats only mydriatic camera systems. The general principles and techniques outlined here apply to both kinds.

The Fundus Camera—Anatomy

The principal parts of the fundus camera that produce the retinal image of the patient's eye for photography are outlined in detail. As with an automobile the "basic" camera requires certain parts. "Extras" increase operator ease and efficiency, but are not required for photographic operation.

Dissection of a generic fundus camera will best illustrate the features necessary for functional operation. User familiarity with each of these features will facilitate the correct use of such a camera.

Common to all ophthalmic photographic systems are the resting supports for the patient, namely the cup for the chin and bar for the forehead, mounted to a table base to stabilize the subject to be photographed (Figure 5.4). The chinrest usually has an adjustment to allow for variations in patient chin to forehead distance. Mounted on top of the forehead rest is a fixation device that moves freely on a double jointed elbow or flex arm to a position in front of either of the patient's eyes to help the patient maintain a fixed direction of gaze. This fixation device can contain a flickering or constant light source of red, white, or green to be more useful.

The table base on which the chinrest is mounted should also be adjustable to fit the various sized persons to be photographed. Various table bases have been designed to allow access by patients in wheelchairs. Manual or electric means of table height adjustment are available.

Also mounted on a movable track on the table base is a camera base mount for the retinal fundus camera unit. This mount should operate like a slit lamp base to allow movement both side-to-side (x-axis) and toward and away (y-axis) from the patient to allow correct camera position. There may be a separate control to raise and lower the camera (z-axis) either by a rotation of the joystick controlling x-y axis movement, or with a separate control to make vertical adjustments (Figure 5.4).

Light Path Into and Out of the Patient's Eye

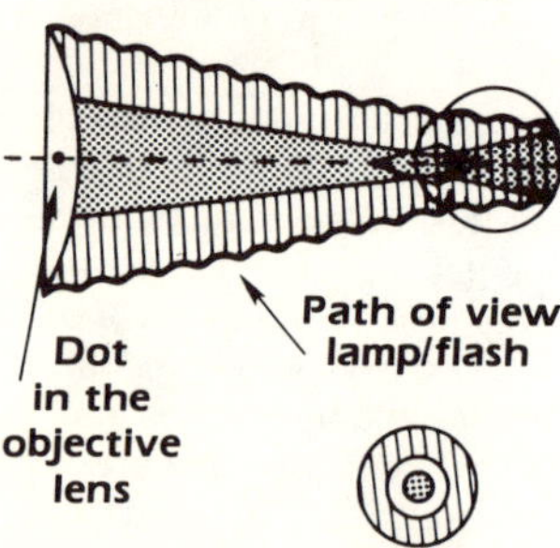

Figure 5.3 The light path of illumination and observation light of the fundus camera first into, then out of, a patient's eye. The dot breaks up the central rays of light, so they are not reflected directly back into the camera lens from the curved surface of the patient's cornea and lens.

Mounted on the camera base is the retinal camera itself. The retinal camera is mounted on a pivot point, coincident with a vertical line descending through the front principal focal point of the objective lens directly to the floor. This mount point facilitates the swinging of the retinal camera from side-to-side on this pivot allowing scanning of patient's retina without moving the base of the camera mount. Often

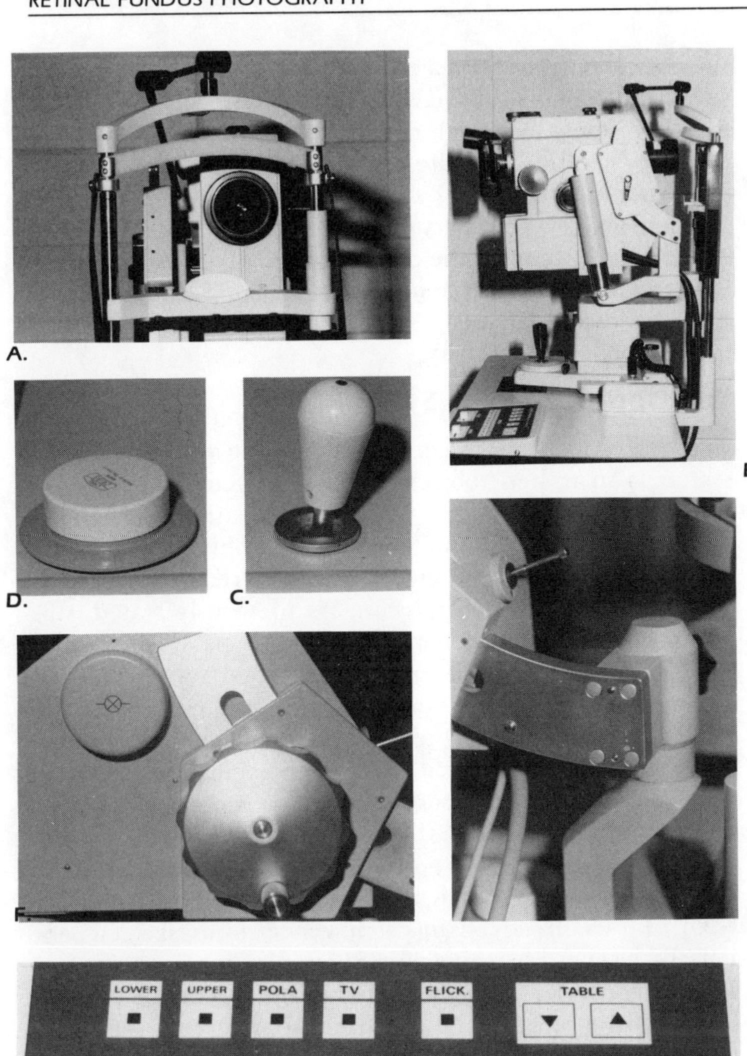

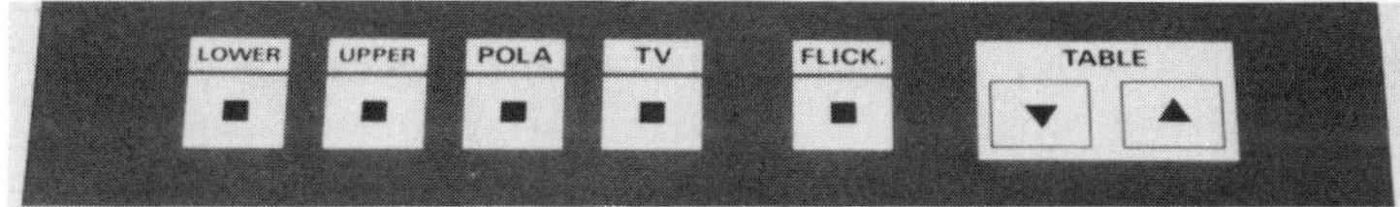

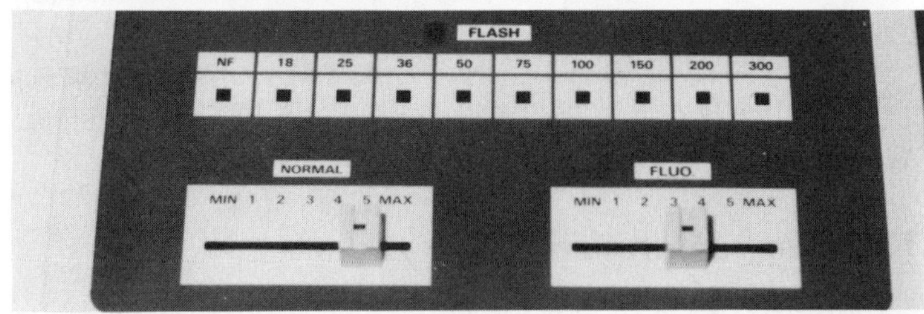

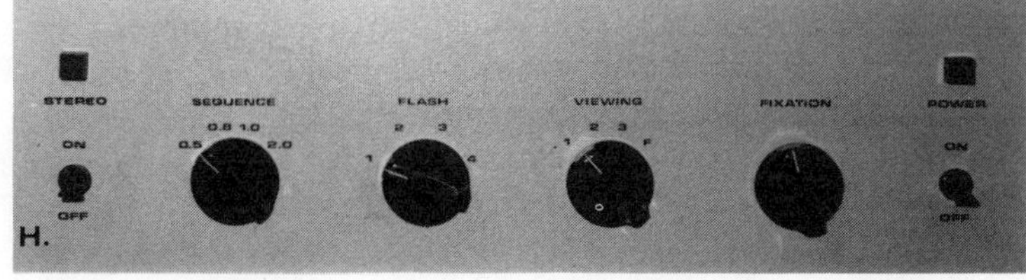

Figure 5.4 Components of the fundus camera support unit and power pack: **A.** Chinrest and fixation device. **B.** Camera base and table. **C.** Joystick. **D.** Vertical adjustment knob. **E.** Pivot mount. **F.** Tilt mechanism. **G.** Power unit control panels for a Topcon. **H.** A Zeiss fundus camera.

the optical head rests on a tilt mechanism that allows vertical swing movements on this same pivot point to examine the patient's upper or lower retina. These camera movement features greatly facilitate rapid performance of retinal photography (Figure 5.4).

There are two necessary parts comprising the optical head of the fundus camera: the optical imaging system, and the illumination exposure system. (Refer to Figure 5.4 for illustration of the components.)

The Optical Imaging System

The first and primary component of the optical imaging system is an aspheric objective lens mounted in a cylindrical tube. When placed in position before the patient, its working distance is only 35–50mm from the eye. This lens is of high optical quality and cost, and is coated to reduce reflections and increase light transmission. As previously stated, this lens serves as an indirect ophthalmoscope, passing light into the patient's eye (a self-contained internal reflector), then gathering the exiting light to focus it within its own central axis as an aerial image. This "telescope"—more correctly "microscope"—passes its reflected image to a point in the "telescope" barrel at which further lenses allow various optical manipulations of the virtual image, that is, corrections for sphere, cylinder, and axis. Beyond this point a simple converging lens passes the aerial image to a SLR 35mm camera back for recording. Such a camera back contains a viewfinder for image composition. By placing a swinging mirror between the converging lens and camera back at a 45° angle, the image rays can be directed up, down, or sideways to a separate eyepiece or secondary camera body. Such a mirror, as in a SLR camera, is introduced or removed from the optical axis during exposure to allow the image to follow the light path desired. Various magnifications palce cameras and viewfinders above, beside, or below at right angles to the principal light axis to facilitate the use of more than one camera body.

The viewlamp, for image composition and focus, and the electronic flash system used to record the image on film share a common path to the patient's eye. In each individual camera system, design location of these two illumination components varies, but both must meet and follow the same path through the objective lens into the patient's eye.

The Illumination Exposure System

The human eye is round; the patient's dilated pupil should be round; so the optimal illumination system should also project a round, cylindrical beam of light into the patient's eye for viewing, focusing, and exposure. Tungsten light bulbs provide view illumination for the fundus camera. This is projected from below the optical axis through a set of converging and diverging lenses and mirrored surfaces to pass outward through the aspheric objective lens and into the patient's eye.

Unaltered, the central ray of this light beam would strike the curved cornea and lens and reflect directly back along the principal axis to the film there, overexposing the film and marring central resolution. To overcome this problem, a black dot is placed within the aspheric lens (Figure 5.3). This dot causes the central ray to project a shadow onto the patient's cornea and lens, surrounded by a ring of illumination passing into the patient's eye. This "donut" of illumination light contains a hollow center or "hole." The reflected light from within the patient's eye exits the eye through the hole, then follows the optical imaging axis to the film plane or photographer's eye.

To demonstrate this "donut," place a piece of white paper perpendicular to the principal axis of the light exiting the objective. Use a millimeter rule to measure the height of the "donut." This distance is the minimum size of the dilated pupil required for any particular retinal fundus camera to operate efficiently.

Placed at a right angle or the same axis of the illumination system is an electronic flash tube used to take photographs (Figure 5.5). The flash illumination follows the same optical path as the view lamp light, entering the eye as a "donut"—exiting through the hole. If the donut hole is within the dilated pupil, but the illumination ring exceeds the pupillary diameter, less light will enter the eye and exit it for exposure. Always check that the patient is adequately dilated for the fundus camera used. Central areas of gray fuzz in your photographs frequently indicate poor dilation.

The eyepiece of the fundus camera, whether separate or part of the 35mm camera back, must be adjustable for the photographer's accommodative error. The camera system is much like a telescope focused on the moon. Accommodation must be completely relaxed while using the instrument to achieve critical focus as the photographer's eye and the film's focal plane must be coincident and both focused on infinity.

Dialing in the photographer's refractive error on the eyepiece prevents the eye from aiding in focusing images by changing the shape of its own lens. Within the eyepiece is a reticule, a network or grid of fine lines dividing the field of view into a series of small squares or wedges (Figure 5.6). Rotate the eyepiece counterclockwise until it stops. This is the extreme plus position. Slowly and continuously rotate this housing clockwise until the network of lines becomes sharp. Do this with both eyes open in a dimly lit or dark room holding a white card in front of the objective lens. Critical image focus on the film plane cannot be achieved without this step. This process eliminates photographer accommodation.

The eyepiece and objective lenses magnify the view, making viewing easier. Supplementary lenses to the optical path

The eyepiece reticule housing frequently comes in direct contact with many photographers' lids and orbital bones. The reticule can be accidentally turned and shifted from the correct setting. A periodic check of this setting should be done. Have the patient close his eye. Use the highly reflective lid surface to recheck the reticule setting during the work day.

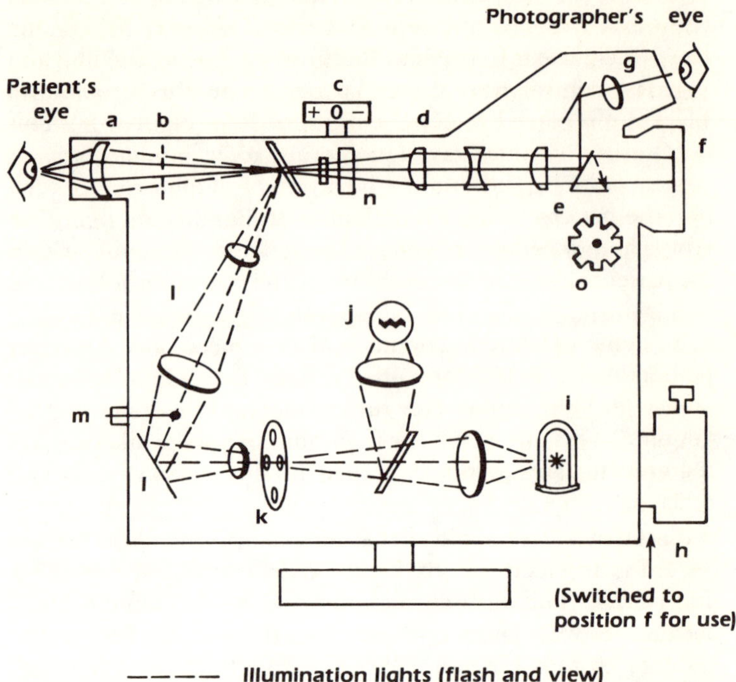

Figure 5.5 Basic components of a fundus camera—Top: (a) objective lens, (b) aerial image in camera, (c) diopter compensator, (d) angle converter, (e) swing mirror, (f) 35mm camera body, (g) separate eyepiece viewfinder, (h) auxiliary camera body, (i) flash tube, (j) view lamp, (k) filter wheel (or slot), (l) optical illumination lenses and mirrors, (m) internal fixation device, (n) filter slide, (o) focus knob. Bottom: Cutaway of a Zeiss fundus camera.

increase either field of view or magnification. These two variables work inversely, that is, as magnification is increased the angle of retina covered is reduced. Conversely, as angle or field of view increases, magnification diminishes. The knob or lever used to select angle of view is called the "angle changer" (Figure 5.7).

Optically each eye viewed will be of varying axial length. A focusing rack moves the camera back and forth in combination with the supplementary converging lens of the camera to properly focus on any individual subject. When the camera focus rack reaches the limits of focus, another lens can be added to the optical system to enable focusing on longer (myopic "−") eyes or shorter (hyperopic or aphakic "+") eyes. This is called the diopter (light bending power) compensation device and is used when the normal (emmetropic) range of axial lengths is exceeded. All these optical mechanisms are contained in a box or shell, the camera body housing.

The camera objective is mounted in a barrel extending toward the patient. A slot can be added in the side of the box or housing to slide filters into the light path either before or after the light enters the patient's eye. The major use of these filters will be treated in the following chapter on fluorescein angiography.

Some cameras also include a fan to cool the viewing lamp, a diaphragm to constrict the illuminating light beam for use on patients with small pupils, and a data recording device for imprinting patient data onto the film in the camera body. These recording devices can be attached to the 35mm camera back or operate inside the fundus camera housing. Patient name and/or number will be recorded on the film with each exposure.

The final component is power. Electricity must light the view bulb and discharge the flash. Wiring will connect the power pack unit with its capacitors, resistors, and so on, to the camera. A means of adjusting view lamp intensity (a rheostat), and a variable flash output control are both mandatory for all but the simplest system.

The previous description is of a generic fundus camera. In today's equipment market, there are more than a half dozen manufacturers of such cameras. All these systems vary the way cars vary, more features on one than another, but they all "get you there," that is, they all contain the basic parts used to take retinal photographs.

There are currently eight major manufacturers of fundus cameras: Canon, Kowa, Mamiya, Nikon, Olympus, Topcon, Carl Zeiss, and Zeiss-Jena (East German). Mamiya and Zeiss-Jena cameras are seldom seen or used in America. Each of the remaining six cameras can produce fine images. Figure 5.8 is a composite of six photographs of my left eye, each one taken with a different fundus camera on the same day by Mark Maio.

Each camera used correctly will take fine photographs. Each of you will be using a different camera. Step one in using a fundus camera is to find the manual that came with the camera and *read it!* Many questions you have will be answered by the manual. If you do not have a manual, write to the manufacturer and request one. Specify the model

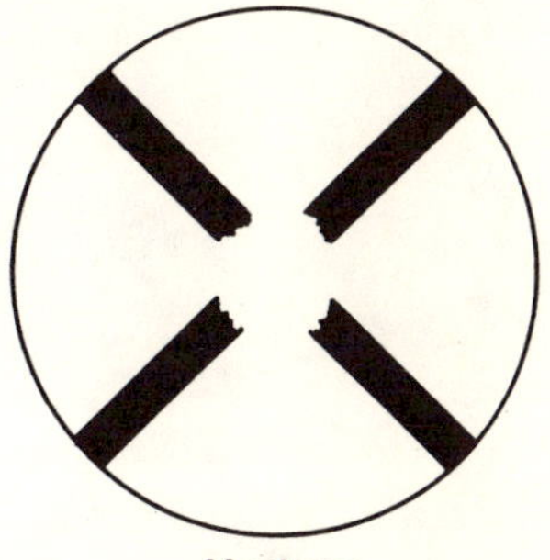

Unsharp reticule

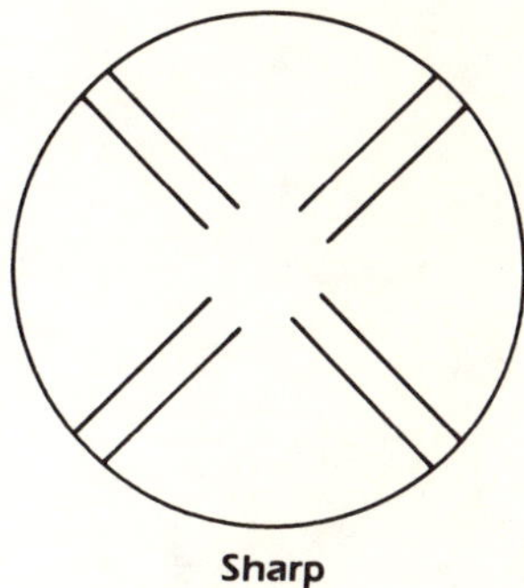

Sharp reticule

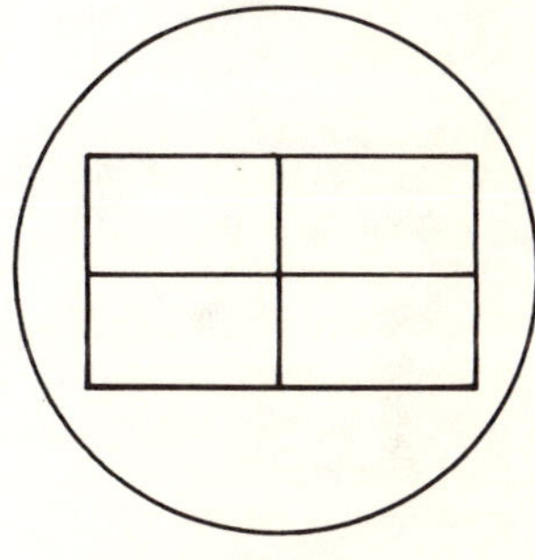

Sharp pattern variation

Figure 5.6 An unsharp reticule (top). The same reticule set correctly (center). A different reticule pattern set correctly (bottom).

Repetition of the dictum—When all else fails, read the directions. Avoid the necessity of applying this rule, by reading the manual first. If questions remain, consult the manufacturer or an experienced ophthalmic photographer.

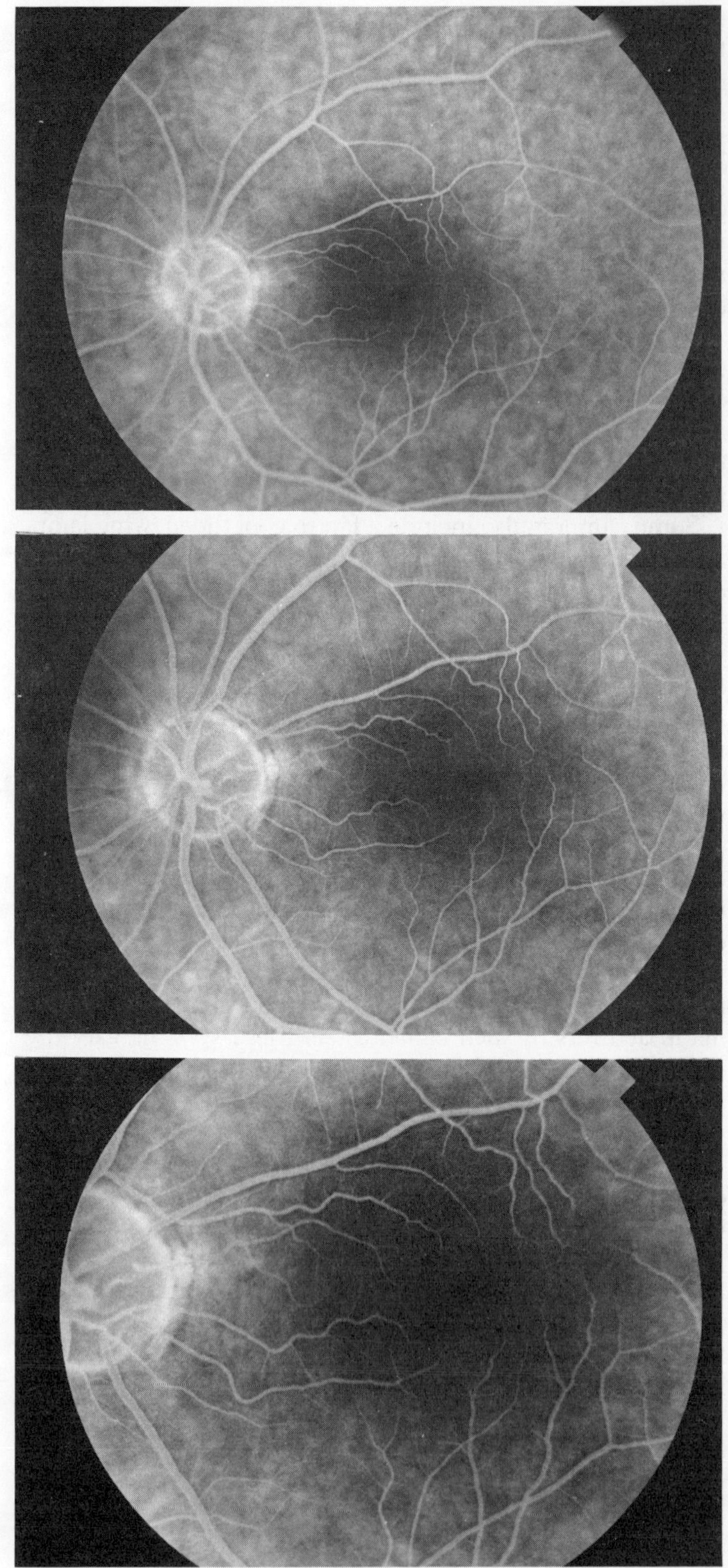

Figure 5.7 Three different angles of view of the same eye during an angiogram: 50° (top), 35° (center), 20° (bottom).

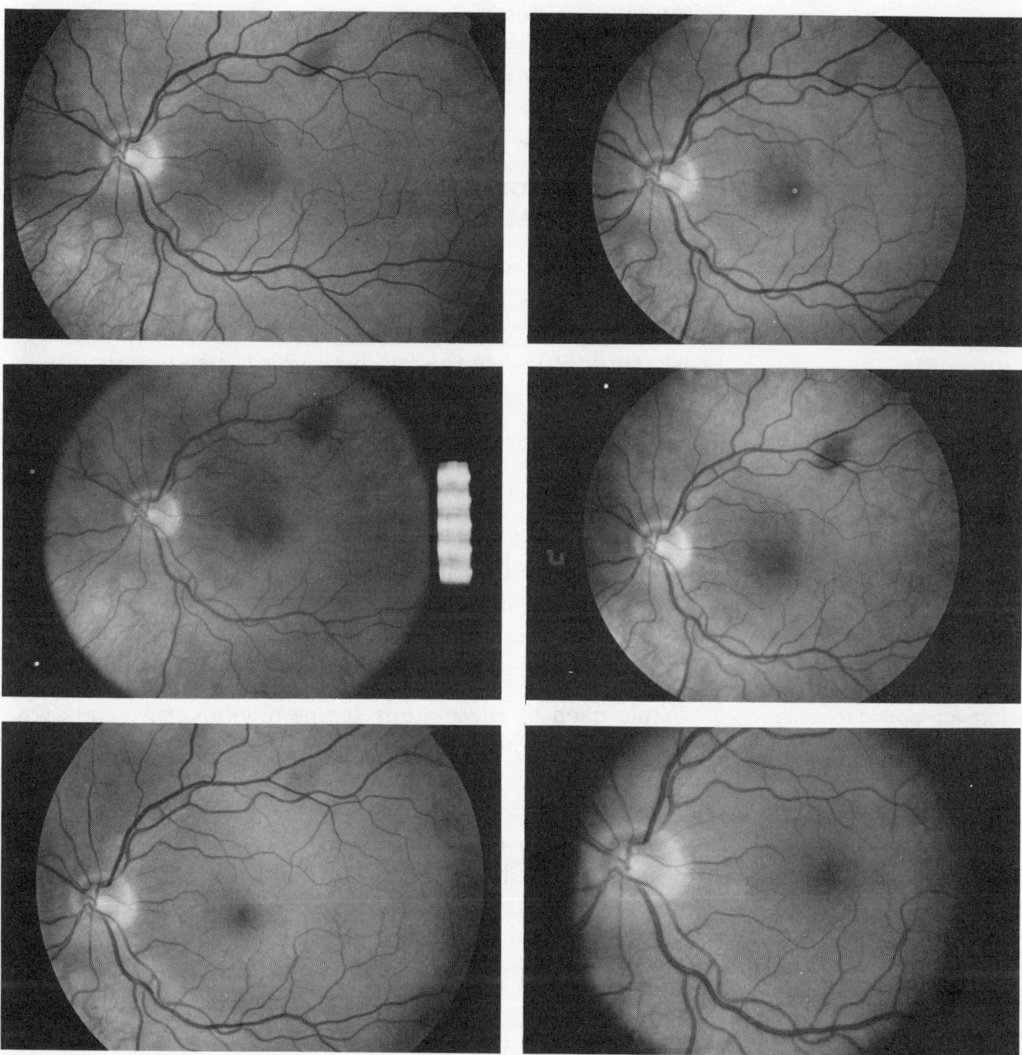

Figure 5.8 The same fundus taken with the six commonly used retinal cameras: Canon 60° (top left), Kowa 45° (top right), Nikon 50° (center left), Olympus 45° (center right), Topcon 50° (bottom left), Zeiss 35° (bottom right).

number of your instrument. The intent of this book is not to analyze each camera in detail. As we saw in the last section, the parts necessary to record images can be modified or placed in various positions but each system must follow basic technical requirements. The methods of photography that follow apply equally to all systems available.

There are other fundus imaging systems for special uses. MIRA makes an ultra-wide (140 °) angle camera. Kowa and Reichert make hand-held fundus cameras. Humphrey Instruments and PAR Technologies, among others, make image digitation systems that store fundus images in a computer and analyze this data. Each of these digital systems still uses the same principles of focusing and collecting light via an optical objective to store data for later viewing and interpretation. Twenty five years ago Dr. Donaldson made the simultaneous stereo camera, some of which are still in use today. This camera and others like it that followed take two simultaneous images. When paired and viewed together, images are seen in three dimensions.

Fundus Photography—Technique and Patient Management

Now that we have seen the design of the camera, and are familiar with its components, let's learn the technique for achieving good, useful images (how to use one)! To teach a basic student to use the fundus camera, begin with:

Preparation for the Day

Before beginning to photograph patients you should:

- be sure that your camera is in working order
- inspect the front objective lens of the camera to ensure that it is clean
- confirm your reticule setting on the camera
- set out the supplies you need

Read these instructions for cleaning the front surface of the camera's objective lens before attempting to clean the lens. Make certain the cleaning solution is appropriate for the camera cleaner combination used. The coating on the lens can be damaged by the wrong cleaning solution.

While each of these steps seems obvious, the stress you will avoid in a busy day by taking 15 minutes to do them before you see your first patient will be ample reward.

The camera should be turned on when you come into the office. Uncover the lens, turn the viewing illumination up, and inspect the lens to see if there is dust, grease or other foreign substances on it. The increased illumination level facilitates inspection and cleaning. Should the lens need cleaning observe the following rules:

Routine dilation for fundus photography requires application of two types of dilating agents, a cycloplegic agent and a mydriatic agent. The mydriatic agent, in 2.5% concentration, causes the dilator muscle of the iris to contract, dilating the pupil. The cycloplegic, usually in 1% concentration, blocks the contraction of the sphincter muscle of the iris as well as relaxing contraction of the ciliary muscle (accommodation), also causing dilation of the pupil. Allow one-half hour to pass after application of the drops for maximum dilation. Two or three applications of drops may be necessary for some patients.

1. Never touch the lens with a finger because skin oil will leave a residue.
2. Never use water to clean the lens. The water will enter the edge of the lens, separate the compound lens elements, and destroy the optics of the system.
3. Never use anything to clean a lens not *specifically* recommended by the manufacturer of your camera. Each camera manufacturer coats (or does not) the front surface of the objective lens differently. Therefore only the manufacturer can recommend the correct cleaning solution to use.
4. Avoid packaged cotton tipped applicators. The glue used to hold on the cotton may melt in the cleaning solution and further dirty the lens. If drastic cleaning is necessary, use absorbent cotton in 16 oz. rolls, and twirl small amounts around the noncottoned end of the applicator. This allows the use of more of the cotton for cleaning and avoids glues.

5. Start with a pneumatic bulb or can of compressed air (avoid canned air if possible). Always attempt to blow foreign objects off the lens from the side across the lens surface. Blowing directly into the lens along the light path only spreads dust and dirt into the edges of the lens.
6. When you must use cleaning solutions,
    a) Put the solution on the cotton applicator or lens tissue, then apply this to the lens.
    b) Start at the center of the lens and *gently* rub in an ever increasing spiral to the edges of the lens.
    c) Once you lift an applicator off the objective lens, discard it and continue with a fresh one.
    d) Cleaners will leave a residue on the lens, so use clean cotton to repeat the spiral to remove it. Then blow the cotton off with the pneumatic bulb.
7. Remember glass is a *soft* surface. Hard rubbing will scratch the surface of the lens, and compromise pictures, not to mention ruin the lens.
8. Remember there is *normally* a black or grey dot in the center of the objective lens to block the central light ray path from eye to film. Don't try to clean it off (some have tried unknowingly and ruined the lens).
9. Cover the lens at all times except when taking pictures. Cleaning the lens is not a rewarding experience. Avoid the problem by preventing exposure to air, dust, and other foreign substances.
10. Do not talk to the patient when the lens is uncovered.

At this point, the lens is clean, the instrument is working—the viewing lamp is on, and no alarm lights show on the power pack. Next you should preset the reticule in the eyepiece of the camera. Hold a white card in front of the objective, turn up the view lamp, rotate the eyepiece from extreme plus clockwise until the fine lines visible in the eyepiece become sharp. Check the scored marks on the rotating lens against the scored line on the stationary eyepiece housing. Note the setting (say +1). Repeat twice more *with both eyes open* to ensure relaxed accommodation. If the setting is similar each time, tape the eyepiece in place to ensure you do not move the eyepiece during the day while taking pictures. The eyepiece set correctly for your eye puts the film plane of the 35mm camera in the same plane of focus as the one you see in the eyepiece when you focus on the patient's fundus. Without this critical setting, though you may focus correctly, the pictures you take will not necessarily be infocus on the film. A camera that is used daily by more than one person will need to have the eyepiece setting constantly changed, as each user will have a different setting. Put an empty film box over the eyepiece when you are not using the camera. This box becomes a reminder to all users to reset the eyepiece before using the camera.

Finally set out the film you will use in a convenient place. Be sure you have an adequate supply available for the day. If doing angiography, load one syringe and set up the IV kit necessary for injection (more in the following chapter). Put a spare view lamp in an easily accessed place in case the one in the camera fails during photography. Know how to change the view bulb on your camera (instructions are in the manual). Use a cloth to remove a burned out bulb, since it will be very hot. Avoid handling the glass part of the new bulb with your fingers to prevent finger oil from penetrating through the glass and diminishing the life of the bulb. Always keep *at least* two spare view lamps and one spare flash tube on hand. Though each has a long life, like tires, they can pop at any time, and without a spare you are waiting beside the road for help to arrive.

While not a daily preparation, a log manual and identification system should be used to keep track of your work. Some camera systems allow the imprinting of patient name or an ID number directly onto the film. Others require the photographer to actually photograph the patient's name on a white card prior to photography. Include on this name tag the patient name, date, chart number and any other relevant data required in your work setting. For example, Jones, M 6/24/86 #361 232 might appear on a tag. This simple photograph between patients fundus slides will facilitate slide sorting and labeling later. Remember, with most fundus cameras you must change the diopter compensation device to + to focus on a hand-held nametag. Return the diopter compensator to 0 immediately after you shoot the nametag, as focusing on the retina will be difficult if not impossible if the compensator is left in the + position. The diopter compensator adds supplementary lenses to the optical path to allow focusing on (−) myopic eyes (long axial length), or (+) hyperopic eyes (short axial length), aphakic patients, external eye photographs, and nametags. Start a logbook in which you record each patient procedure sequentially. Log the date, eye, type of photography, diagnosis, and referring physician to facilitate record keeping and avoid mislabelling work. The log method and nametag system should all work for you.

Consult the patient's chart to confirm the photographs the ophthalmologist is requesting.

You are now ready for the actual photo procedure that starts with dilation.

Dilation

The importance of the patient having well dilated pupils cannot be overstressed. The typical orders for dilation are 1% Mydryacil and 2 ½% Neosynephrine applied in a series once to each eye, Neosynephrine first, then Mydryacil a minute later. Maximal dilation will take 20-30 minutes. Before dilating a patient, ***always check*** the patient's chart for contraindications for for dilation, or instructions to use or avoid certain drugs. When in doubt, ask the doctor. A *minimal* dilation of 4–5 millimeters is necessary to achieve satisfactory imagery. A 6–8mm pupil size makes photography much easier. Don't rush dilation. Allow 20–30 minutes for the drops to take full effect. Check the pupils with a penlight to see if the patient's pupils constrict. If so, wait. If not, proceed with fundus photography.

Some patients will come to the camera already dilated. Always check their pupils for constriction, as the patient may have been dilated for some time, and the drops may be wearing off. Stop and reinforce dilation before proceeding. (Use the dilating time to explain the test to the patient.)

Before proceeding to photograph a patient, a plan of action and a description of what is to be done is necessary. The patient's chart and/or the photo request form should provide this information (Figure 5.9). While every retinal photographer may not be familiar with the diseases to be photographed, he or she should have at hand written information about the eye(s) to be photographed, the area(s) of principal interest, and for angiography, the field of view requested for photographing dye transit through arteries and veins. In the office, this information should be written in the chart and available to the photographer prior to seeing the patient. Always read the chart first, and if the information you seek is not there, ask the doctor. If you photograph patients on a referral basis, you may have a photo request form that provides dilation instructions, diagnosis, fields to be photographed, angle of view (20,30,50,60 degree) to be used, referring physician, and so on (Figure 5.9). This form may also include a drawing of the retina on which the area of interest is circled. Any format is useful provided you get the information you need to photograph the patient correctly.

Check to see if previous photographs have been done (by you or someone else). Retrieve these pictures and look at them. Often these pictures will give you a good indication of how easy or difficult the patient may be to photograph. Frequently on the second visit a patient will understand the procedure and cooperate more (or less)!

Follow a plan for consistently recording similar areas of all patients photographed, either the one listed here or one suited to the requirements of the doctor ordering the photography.

Study the photographs too for composition and fields of

A.

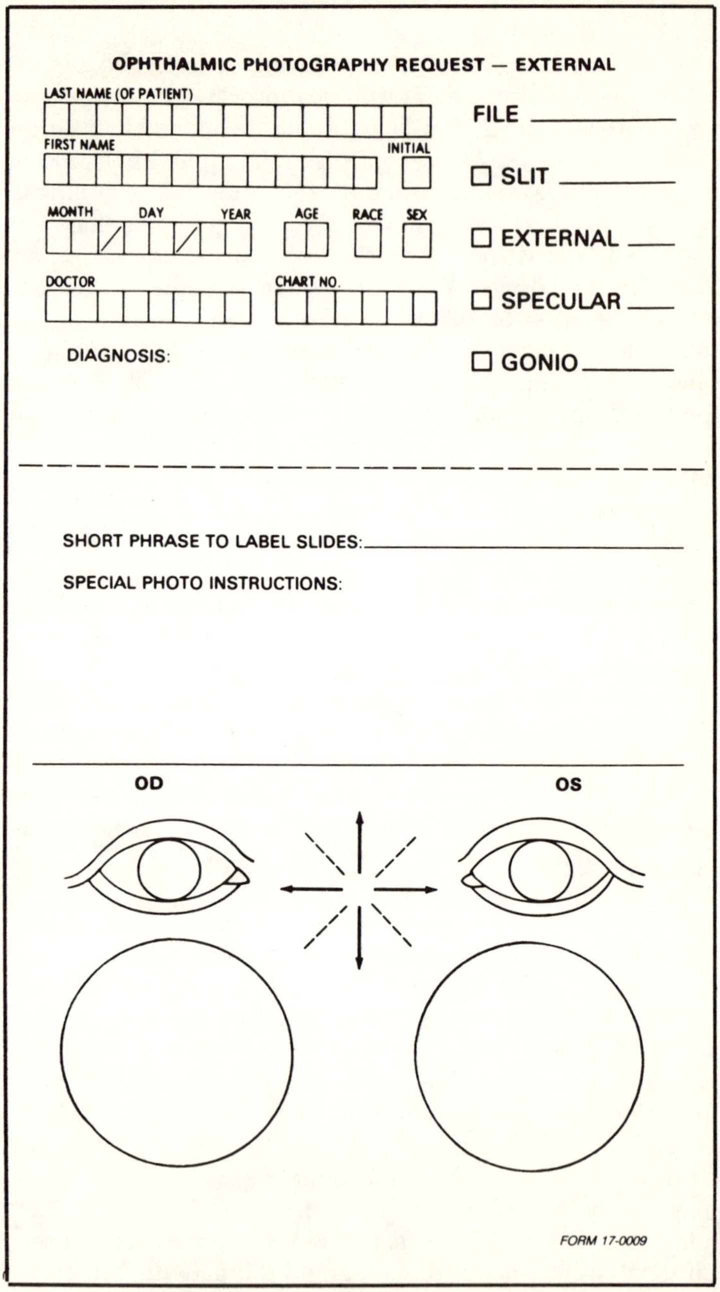

OPHTHALMIC PHOTOGRAPHY REQUEST — EXTERNAL

LAST NAME (OF PATIENT)

FIRST NAME INITIAL

MONTH DAY YEAR AGE RACE SEX

DOCTOR CHART NO.

DIAGNOSIS:

FILE ____

☐ SLIT ____

☐ EXTERNAL ____

☐ SPECULAR ____

☐ GONIO ____

SHORT PHRASE TO LABEL SLIDES: ____

SPECIAL PHOTO INSTRUCTIONS:

OD OS

FORM 17-0009

Mark Maio

Figure 5.9 A. A photo request form for external and slit lamp photography.

view. Attempt to reproduce the same areas of interest in the new set of pictures you are about to take. Comparison of photographs from visit to visit is greatly facilitated when the same field of view recurs regularly, as when following a tumor. If improvement is possible, do so by all means.

B.

THE EMORY CLINIC
Section of Ophthalmology
REQUEST FOR FLUORESCEIN FUNDUSCOPIC STUDIES

DATE TO BE PHOTOGRAPHED ________ DILATE WITH: (SPECIFY DRUG) ________

PATIENT'S NAME ________ AGE ________ STAFF PHYSICIAN (OR PHYSICIAN TO INTERPRET STUDY) ________

CHART # ________ PATIENT REFERRED BY ________

HISTORY AND CLINICAL FINDINGS:

VISUAL ACUITY: OD

VISUAL ACUITY: OS

Camera: _____ Zeiss _____ Canon

_____ Kodachromes and Fluorescein Angiogram
_____ Kodachromes Only
_____ Series
_____ 2X

_____ Stat Negs By ________
_____ Call Patient:
Date ________
Time ________
Phone ________
_____ Return for PCA ________
_____ Send letter ________
_____ Compare old photos ________

FA Information:
Transit Phase Photos: OD OS
Late Pictures_____ 5 min. _____ Other
Patient has had previous FA study?
_____ No _____ Yes _____ Here
_____ Other ________

INDICATE AREAS TO BE PHOTOGRAPHED

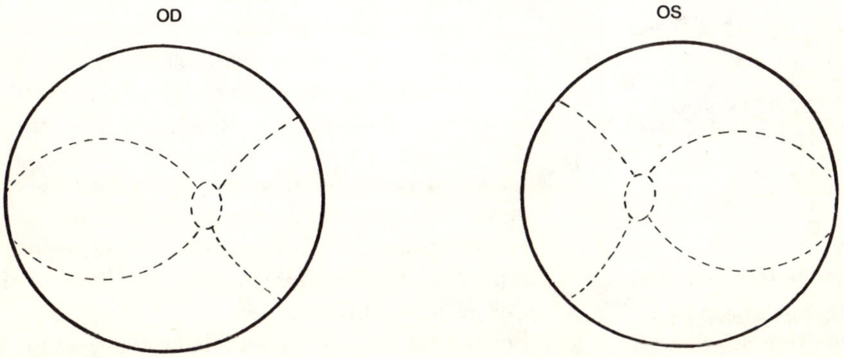

OD OS

PHOTOGRAPHER'S COMMENTS:

FORM 17 0005

Mark Maio

Figure 5.9 B. Example of a photo request form for fundus photography and fluorescein angiography.

The Photo Plan

Each doctor will want certain photographs taken of each patient. Reading the chart will provide some of the medical information you need to get the right pictures.

A regular pattern of photography of every patient will always give you reliable, consistent information on every patient. You need a regular photo plan. Here is a suggestion:

- First Field OD—optic disc centered (stereo pair optional)
- Second Field OD—macula centered (stereo pair optional)
- Third Field OD—other areas of interest (diabetic survey, areas of vascular occlusion, peripheral retina diseases, tumors, and so on).

These views can be at either 35° angle or 50°. In the macula, it is best to take a 30–35° view. Then repeat on the left eye the same pattern; optic disc centered, macula, and other areas of interest.

If for any reason you return to the other eye again *always* shoot the macula first including in this picture a portion of the optic disc, to ensure correctly labeling the pictures that follow.

While it is outside the scope of this book to explain retinal disease, certain common diseases need special photographs for diagnosis and/or treatment. They are:

1. Diabetic survey. Seven overlapping fields which document the entire posterior pole especially the four arcades of blood vessels exiting and reentering the optic disc (Figure 5.10).
2. Vascular occlusive disease (blocked arteries and veins). Document the extent of the changes out to the periphery. With central vein occlusions, take a representative picture in each quadrant of the midperipheral retina.
3. Peripheral retinal disease. Take representative pictures in all quadrants affected (e.g., retintis pigmentosa, Coates disease, sickle cell retinopathy, etc.).
4. Tumors. Center the tumor in the frame. If the tumor exceeds the frame edges, start at the superior margin and document its edges in sequential photographs clockwise until you return to the starting point.
5. Glaucoma. Take stereo disc photos (see Stereo section) plus a macula shot at 35° or higher magnification.

Thoroughly read a book or section from a text on retinal anatomy to become familiar with the structures of the retina and its vascular systems. To help describe areas of pathology, the retina is divided into four quarters or quadrants. A straight line drawn horizontally through the optic disk and fovea divides the retina into superior and inferior portions. A straight line drawn vertically through the optic disk divides the retina into nasal and temporal portions. A request form or chart will indicate the area to be photographed is in, for example, the superior nasal quadrant of the left eye.

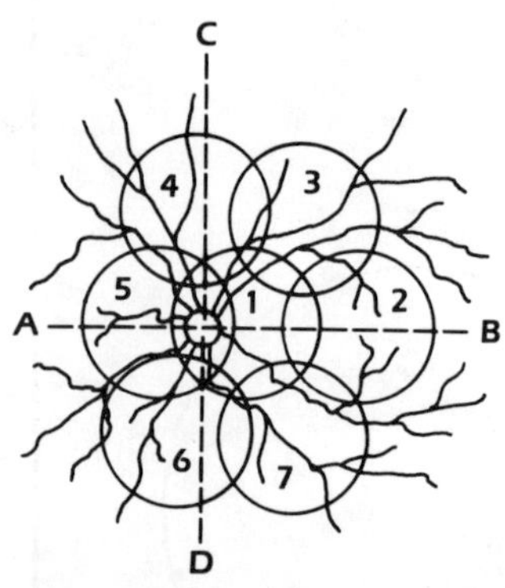

OS (oculus sinister—: left eye)

The broken lines divide the retina into four quadrants: AB superior-inferior; CD nasal-temporal.

Figure 5.10 Seven overlapping fields of view commonly used to document diabetic retinal disorders, as well as other retinal conditions. The broken lines divide the retina into four quadrants—AB superior-inferior, CD nasal-temporal.

6. Macular diseases. Stereo the macula; also photograph the disc too in stereo at a 35° field setting.

When taking fundus photographs, take the extra minute necessary to neatly compose an image. Center the area of interest and focus the camera in this area, not at the edge of the picture. You are using a microscope with very fine levels of focus.

Focus on the layer of the pathology to be photographed. Retinal pigment, for example, is at a deeper level than sensory retinal blood vessels, so change the focus knob to correctly image the level you wish to appear in focus.

Use the fundus camera to photograph the external front surfaces of the eye—especially to document poor patient dilation and/or media opacities that compromise photographic quality.

Corneal edema and cataracts can impair your ability to focus on and photograph a patient's eye with either of these conditions. Take an external picture of these media opacities for reference and to demonstrate the optical limits in these patients. Pull the fundus camera back away from the patient. Change the diopter setting to (+) or external plus (+).

Focus on the cornea (or lens) and take a picture. File this with the retinal fundus photos. The external photo will explain quickly and clearly to anyone examining the patient's photos the physical limitations that the patient's eye created for the photographer.

Fundus photographs taken after a gonioscopic lens has been applanated to the cornea will be less clear than normal. When possible, ask the doctor to allow photography before gonioscopic exams. When this is not possible, irrigate the patient's eye with a solution that contains calcium to avoid corneal dehydration. This will clear the cornea temporarily and improve focus. Reapply the solution between each 2–3 pictures to keep the cornea clear.

To photograph a cataract or other lens opacity, use the same plus (+) diopter setting (Figure 5.11). Frame the dilated pupil in the center of the eyepiece. Adjust focus onto the lenticular (lens) opacities. Shift the patient's fixation so the optic disc of the eye being photographed is directly behind the lens. The background will appear yellow, rather than orange, and act to transilluminate the media opacities more effectively while taking such a picture. You will also be able to observe the area of the lens through which the fundus appears most clear. Use this area to project the light beam for photography into the retina when you shift the camera back into position to photograph the fundus. Pictures of compromised media will document these changes and demonstrate to anyone looking at the fundus photos the difficulty encountered taking them (Fig. 5.11).

Above all don't be guilty of the WNL syndrome—WNL conventionally means "within normal limits." In fundus photography it means "we never looked." Use the camera to

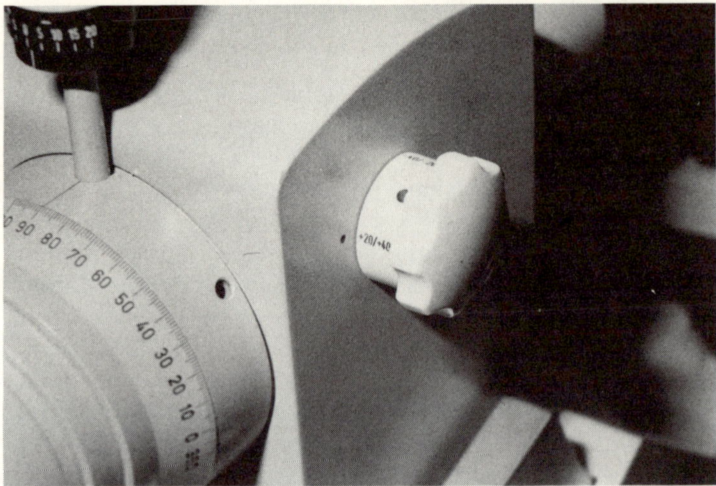

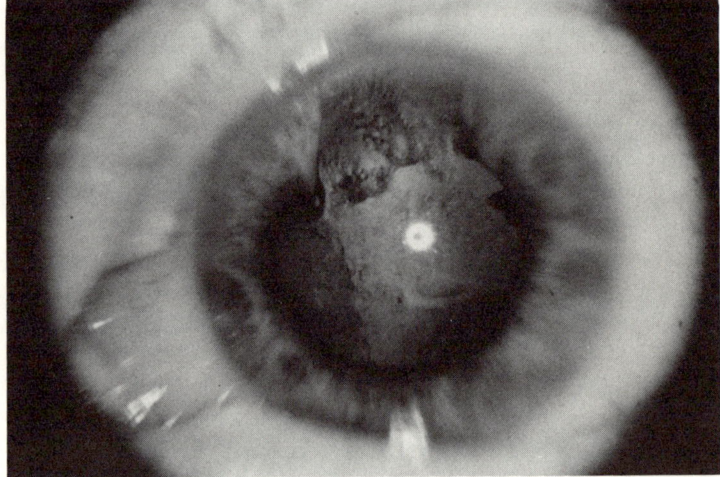

Figure 5.11 A diopter compensation wheel on the Zeiss FF3 retinal camera (top). A photograph of anterior segment pathology taken with the same fundus camera (bottom).

scan the retina. There *is* more back there than the disc and the macula.

When the photographer is educated about the patient's eye, the photographer should now educate the patient about the photographic procedure.

Patient Education

There are three variables in every situation when fundus photography is necessary: the patient, the camera, and the photographer. The patient must remain the centerpiece. The patient's cooperation is 50% of the effort. Spend two or three minutes explaining the procedure to each patient. Keep an 11 × 14 color photograph on your desk to show each patient what the retina looks like and what we will be doing ("no, not x-rays"). Even the $^{20}/_{400}$ patient appreciates some detail in such a picture. The picture and the explanation relieve some of the patient's anxiety. We constantly see patients with compromised vision who may fear they are going blind. By empathizing and explaining we can win the patient's confidence. The more the patient cooperates, the better our photographs. Tell the patients: "The doctor has asked me to take some photographs inside your eyes. With this special camera I have here I can look through your dilated pupils and see into the back of your eyes. This camera can then take color photographs, which when developed the doctor can examine to determine what is occurring inside your eyes."

Patient Positioning

Having explained the procedure, position the patient in the chin rest. Adjustable pneumatic stools are a great aid to quickly adjust for patient height, as well as yours. A rug under the camera area will keep stool movement to a minimum. Keep the patient's (and your) spine erect, not bent. Make sure the patient is positioned so the forehead leans slightly forward onto the forehead rest bar. Achieve this by slightly elevating the patient's posterior (buttocks) on the stool. Gravity will keep the patient leaning forward and down, and prevent the patient from drawing away from the camera. This same technique works for positioning the patient of large girth. Arm rests are nice but not necessary. Patient comfort is a critical part of taking the photograph.

Patient comfort speeds up photography. Remember the patient is seeing you for only a few minutes. The patient's concern for his or her vision may be a barrier to communication and cooperation during photography. Practice patience with the patient. Reassure with physical and verbal contact. Encourage even poor efforts by the patient.

When the patient's head is placed in the chin rest, adjust the chin bar up or down so the patient's forehead rests on the upper rest. All these maneuvers should be done by the photographer from a position at the side of the camera near the patient. Patient positioning is pictorial composition. Set up the picture, then go to the camera to view the subject. Let the patient sit with eyes closed. Center the instrument, that is, adjust the camera's position up/down, in/out, side to side so movement in each direction is possible. Move the entire unit first to a position in front of the patient's right eye. Uncover the lens and project the smallest donut of light possible onto the patient's lid (Figure 5.12). You are now grossly in position, and can move from the side of the camera to the rear eyepiece. Recover then lens for a moment, and have the patient open both eyes. Introduce the fixation target to the patient's left eye. Ask "what do you see?". Let the patient describe to you the light. Learn the patient's visual limits by switching this device to the right eye, and again asking if the patient sees the same light. Patients with central visual impairment will often "see" the light at the edge of their scotoma or blind spot. This noncentral fixation will be erratic and shift the patient's fixation constantly. Be warned by this to avoid using the device

Two useful pieces of equipment are adjustable chairs for the patient and the photographer.

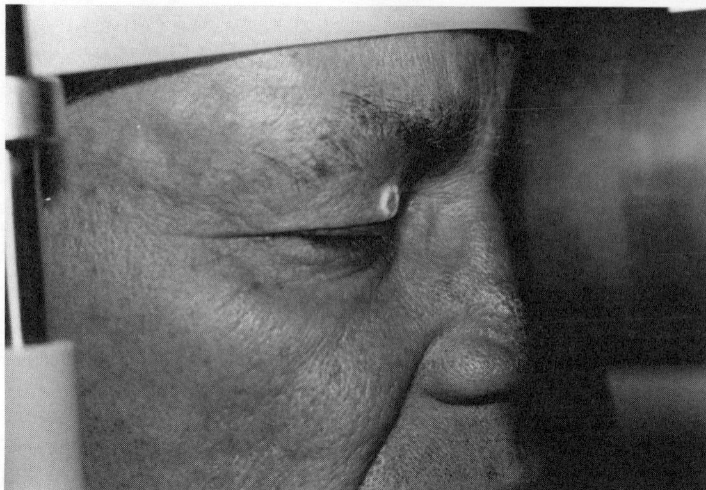

Figure 5.12 The illumination "donut" projected on the closed lid of a patient (right). A correctly positioned camera projects the entire donut through the patient's pupil. The resulting images will be evenly illuminated from edge to edge (bottom left). Improper position will produce unevenly saturated images or vignetting (bottom right).

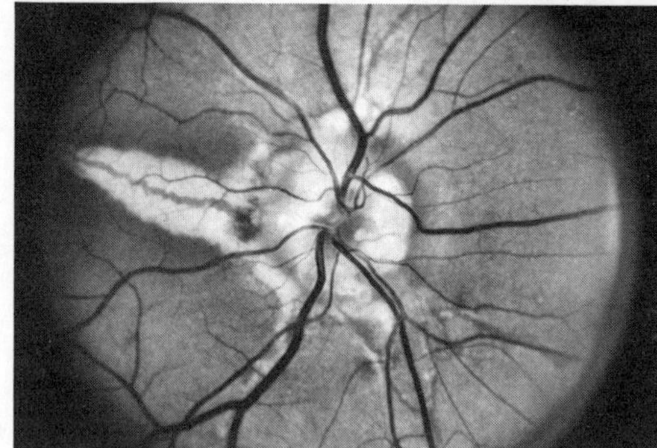

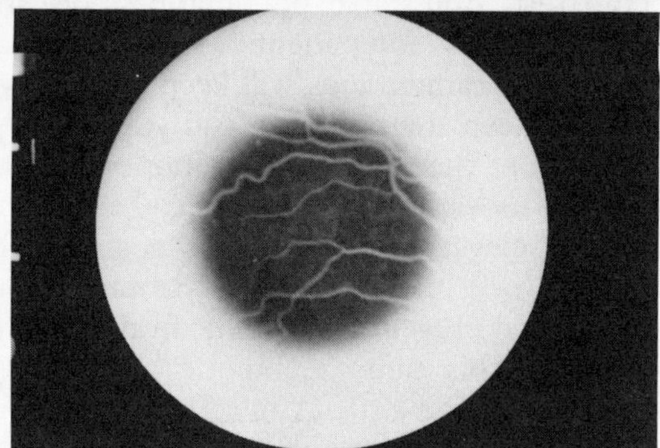

to fixate for stereo pair photos or angiography. Have the patient look in only one fixed direction.

The external fixation device an aid for composition and field definition, not a part of the camera exposure mechanism. Thus its use is voluntary only. An internal fixation device is also usually part of your fundus camera. This device is a needle-like pin with a small ball at the end. By pushing it in somewhere in the optical path, the "pointer" becomes visible to anyone looking into the objective (front) lens of the camera. This device can guide the patient to a fixed position usually only within the immediate optic disk and macular region. The device is visible in the camera eyepiece and appears on film, obscuring the area over which it sits. Thus removing it immediately after guiding a patient to a particular position is desirable. Tell the patient to follow the pointer to a fixed position, then hold that line of sight, while you remove the pointer and take a picture. With practice this method works well for the one-eyed patient as well as those with little or no vision in the other eye.

A variety of techniques are helpful for guiding the patient's fixation to the point which yields the desired field of view in the photograph. Pick the method suited for the limits of the particular patient you are photographing.

Another simple fixation method is as follows: describe the circle of light of the objective lens to the patient as a conventional clock. Ask the patient to look at the center of the clock where the two hands meet (the middle of the light). Observe the fundus. In this position the macula is centered in the eyepiece. Ask the patient to look to the 9 o'clock position of the clock at the edge of the circle. In the right eye this will center the optic disc (in the left gaze at 3 o'clock to center the disk). By guiding the patient around the edges of the clock you can visualize the entire back third of the retina. Even blind or severely compromised individuals see the circle of light and are familiar with a clock. To gain views more peripheral, guide the patient beyond the edge of the circle into the meridian (hour of the clock) of interest.

A word about the external fixation devices and binocular vision is necessary. The two eyes in most individuals move in concert with each other. Thus if you move the external fixation device in any direction, both the patient's eyes follow it *in the same direction* (usually). The fundus camera operates in the same manner and should move in concert in equal amounts in the same direction as the fixation device.

Whenever you move the fixation device up, down or sideways, move the fundus camera in the same direction up, down or sideways.

When shifting fields of view follow the fixation device up, down, or sideways with the fundus camera. Many photographers overlook this obvious mirroring of binocular vision, and get lost quickly, when they change fields (from discto macula, for example). Finally, when fixation is difficult to achieve move the camera only to change fields. The up/down and tilt and swing mechanisms will allow movement to other areas if the patient's gaze remains fixed in one direction. Practice these methods with your patients. Modify any mode to what works for you.

We now have a primed, positioned, fixated patient sitting at the fundus camera. We have positioned the camera so the view light is projected on the closed lid of our patient's eye. We ask the patient to open both eyes, and we readjusted position so the entire beam of light is projected into the patient's eye. This is more easily checked by viewing from the side of the camera, than through its eyepiece. Develop and ingrain the habit of looking at the camera setup and patient from beside, not behind, the camera. Lean out to check where you and the patient are, and to talk to the patient. Don't make the fundus camera a barrier between you. Positioning errors and patient movement are much easier to see and correct from the side vantage, especially for basic level photographers.

Now we achieve correct position and through the eyepiece we see red lines and an orange and yellow background. Using the joystick or control lever, very slightly move in/out, up/down, and back and forth looking for good, even image color saturation—even color across the field we are viewing (Figure 5.12). When we are correctly positioned in all three dimensions, focus the image we see with the focus knob,

What you see in the eyepiece is what will appear on the film. Poor positioning, a dirty lens, drooping lids or yellow crescents must all be eliminated before taking a picture.

then fire the camera to record the image. Ask the patient to blink once before firing to clear the tear film, and open the lids widely. Take a series of predetermined views, then shift to the fellow eye and repeat the pattern.

Well, you ask, how do I know I'm in the right position? The answer is that there are optical clues in the eyepiece. What you see in the eyepiece is what you get on the film.

If the camera is too close or too far from the patient's eye, the beam of light can strike the iris and diffuse the return beam, causing a blue-white haze at the edge of the image to appear in the eyepiece (oversaturation). If the camera is too far away, a whitish haze will result centrally (undersaturation). Reposition after leaning out and looking to see where you are. Often the patient has moved back, away from the light. Reposition the patient or camera as necessary.

When the camera is the correct distance in and and out but slightly off center entering the pupil, a light yellow crescent (like a new crescent moon) will appear at the edge of the frame. *Always* move the camera in the diametrically opposite direction to remove this artifact. If the crescent is on the left side, move right; if it is upper left, move down and right. This crescent is a reflection caused by the outer edge of the view light striking the inner edge of the dilated iris. Remember we are projecting a donut of light into the circular pupil. If dilation is only equal to or smaller than the diameter of the view light beam, we will get reflected light which will compromise our ability to record useful images.

Several rules and suggestions that will facilitate fundus photography follow:

Read and reread the adjacent list of rules and suggestions to ensure good consistent cooperation from your patients. These habits will produce good consistent photographs.

1. Remember, always check dilation when positioning patients. See that the pupil is 6mm plus whenever possible, and holding. When dilation is inadequate or the drops are wearing off, reapply drops and wait 5–10 minutes.
2. Use the minimum level of viewing illumination necessary to see and focus your subject.
3. Don't allow anyone else who is not absolutely necessary in the photo room—distractions are to be avoided. A translator for language barriers is recommended.
4. Allow (encourage) the patient to blink frequently—a wet tear film on the cornea facilitates good focus. Remember, the paitent's eye is a part of the optical system you are using.
5. Encourage the patients to blink just before each picture, then ask them to open wide and hold until the flash. Take the picture immediately after the blink.

6. Allow the patient to rest when necessary.
7. When switching to the other eye, allow the patient to view the camera viewing lamp for approximately 30 seconds to adjust to the intensity of the view lamp. Patients often state the light seems brighter when presented to the second eye to be photographed.
8. Encourage the patient.
9. When cooperation breaks down, STOP and tell the patient to sit back. Reemphasize the importance of the procedure to the patient—then begin again.
10. If eyelids are a problem (not open enough) allow the patient to hold his own eyelid before attempting to do this yourself. Sit the patient back. Ask the patient to close his eyes, then bring his hand up to his right eye lid. Using his index finger, gently lift up the lid immediately above the eye lashes. The removal of the lid and lashes from the light path will usually clear the field of view. The involuntary spasm of lid closure induced by another person holding the lid will be eased or eliminated when the patient holds his own lid. This technique allows easy viewing of the inferior portion of the fundus usually obscured by lids and lashes when the patient is looking down. When necessary hold the lid yourself with a Q-tip or finger, as some patients cannot hold their own lids.
11. As a last resort, get someone else in the office to hold the patient's lids. Teach them the same lid holding technique just outlined. Have the lid holder use the other hand to gently hold the back of the patient's head in the headrest. Allow frequent blinks.
12. Maintain control with the patient. Be gentle but firm with your instructions.
13. Discourage conversation while taking pictures.
14. Watch out for the patient who opens his mouth when he opens his eyes, thus shifting the position of the pupil upward. Tell the patient, "Close your mouth and open your eyes." You will have to repeat this instruction frequently.
15. Speak loud and clear. Many patients' ears do not hear properly either.

Managing The Unusual Patient

When photographing children, have the patient stand rather than sit. Be gentle but firm. Make a game of the procedure. Sacrifice quantity for quality. Keep both parents out of the room (one only if necessary). Talk to the child for a few extra

Photographing the unusual patient will tax the photographer's imagination and patience. For every rule or suggestion there will be more exceptions. Firmness with one individual will work better than with the next. Manners count. A professional attitude should always be displayed.

minutes before beginning. Talk to the child, not the parent. Treat the child as an equal. Don't stop frequently. Set up a field of view and shoot. Avoid constant realignment as much as possible.

For the short patient, lower the camera and raise the stool. Keep a box in the photo room for the patients to set their feet on for stability. For the round or large patient, raise the patient's stool excessively and let the patient fall forward into the chin rest. Gravity will keep the patient in place. For the wheelchair patient, lower the camera and bring the patient forward in the wheelchair. Place a triangular block (like a tire chock) behind the wheels of the chair. This will tip the patient forward from the waist up and keep the patient in contact with the chin rest. Allow frequent rest intervals. For the photophobic patient (everyone's favorite) teach the patient to hold the lids. Use a cotton tip applicator to roll the lid up. Sternly reinforce the need for cooperation. Get help from someone in the office. If all else fails use the view lamp trick.

At the first sign of noncooperation, ask the patient to close both eyes. Turn the view lamp of the camera up to maximum. Proceed to focus on the patient's retina. Explain the bright light is only necessary to establish "initial" focus. Tell the patient, "If you will cooperate for 10 seconds, I will be able to reduce the view lamp intensity significantly. Focus, then reduce viewlamp intensity back to the normal setting, while the patient's eyes are still open. Most patients will markedly increase their level of cooperation. The secret is, of course, to give a little to get a little. Treat this procedure as a special personal favor to the patient (an idea which is universally true). You know you have succeeded when the patient says afterwards, "That wasn't so bad after all."

Camera Maintenance

Know the routine maintenance procedures necessary to keep the fundus camera operational. We have previously discussed optical maintenance (objective lens cleaning). Clean the camera's eyepiece regularly too!

Electrical Maintenance

Know how to change the view lamp, the flash tube, and the fuses in the power supply unit. Most cameras come with a spare view lamp and fuses. The flash tube is expensive, but a spare on hand is highly recommended. Read the camera manual to learn correct removal and installation of lamp, flash and fuses. Keep a record of when the flash tube was installed when replacing one. Make a note in the photo log with red ink. Inspect the flash tube for wear periodically.

The gas inside gradually diminishes with use, building a grey deposit on the inside. Review slides and negatives for gradual loss of density. Color slides will appear darker as the flash tube wears out. Photograph a patient with the old tube, then put in the new one and rephotograph the patient. Inspect the slides when processed to see if there is a significant difference in color saturation. If so replace the old tube with the new or increase the flash setting on the power pack to compensate for this until the old tube wears out. Then replace it. Check with the manufacturer to see if the old flash tube holder can be traded in on a new one. Avoid attempts to repair malfunctions in the power pack. The capacitors carry enough voltage to kill you.

The scheduled maintenance of the fundus camera will produce a long, healthy life for your fundus camera. Don't ignore maintenance.

Schedule an annual maintenance for your camera by a service representative. Have the moveable gears lubricated. Have the internal mirrors cleaned. Do not remove the side plate from the camera to expose the inside to air. Dust may settle on mirrors and lenses, and cause picture artifacts. If necessary have the rear surface of the objectives cleaned. Dust inside the camera settles here too.

Sealed objectives should only be cleaned by the manufacturer's repair personnel.

Clean the camera backs holding the 35mm film regularly. Dust and debris from the constant transit of film through the camera accumulates there. Open the empty camera back and remove this with moist cotton tipped applicators.

Don'ts of Maintenance

Silly as some of these suggestions sound, they are here because some people have done them (and you know who you are)!

1. Do not clean the lens with soap or water.
2. Do not attempt even routine maintenance with the power on.
3. Do not grasp the viewlamp unless it has cooled, or you are wearing a cotton glove, or using a clean hand towel, because you will burn yourself.
4. Do not attempt to repair the power back. The capacitors inside carry enough voltage to kill you. (If you must fix a broken power pack I recommend you turn off the power unit, wait 30 seconds for capacitors to drain then pull the plug out before opening the power pack to allow the capacitors to fully drain.) When the problem is not the view lamp, the flash tube, or a blown fuse, (usually located in the rear of the power supply unit) seek professional help. A blown fuse, like a blown view lamp, will have a broken filament inside. Replace the fuse with one of equal amperage. The fuse's

amperage is usually written on the power unit under the fuse slot. Use slow blow fuses; if recommended by the manufacturer.

5. Do not attempt optical alignment unless you know what you are doing. Even if you think you do, be very cautious adjusting an optical element. Leave it to the manufacturer's service technicians.
6. Do not be afraid to admit you can't solve the problem. Call the manufacturer for help with serious or unknown problems.

Summary

(Step-by-Step) Technique for Fundus Photography

Your own step by step method will vary with practice and depend also on the model fundus camera you use.

1. Prepare for the day ahead. Check the camera; check the eyepiece setting. Set out the supplies you will use this day.
2. Obtain the chart(s) or request forms for the patients to be photographed. Read them.
3. Review any previous photographs the patient may have had done.
4. Explain the test to new (and return) patients.
5. Dilate the patient as instructed.
6. Turn on the camera and set the flash intensity to the correct setting.
7. Photograph the patient's name tag with + diopter setting. Return diopter compensation wheel to 0 (zero) setting immediately.
8. Position the patient comfortably at the camera.
9. Introduce the fixation light to the patient.
10. Have the patient close both eyes.
11. Bring the camera into position in front of the right eye while still seated beside the patient.
12. Fine tune camera position. Project the smallest possible circle of light onto the patient's lid.
13. Have the patient open both eyes and look at the fixation device.
14. Move to camera eyepiece.
15. Establish the initial field of view.
16. Compose the image, focus and shoot.
17. Complete photo documentation in the right eye.
18. Allow the patient to rest.
19. Switch the camera and fixation light positions.
20. Reposition the patient.
21. Repeat steps 12-17 in the left eye.
22. Prepare for angiography or help the patient to the next stop in the clinic or office.

Three Final Points on Technique:

1. The patient will see lights and colors for a few minutes after the pictures are completed. Allow one or two minutes of recovery time before moving the patient off the chair or stool.
2. Empathize with the patient. Have someone photograph your retina. Be the patient. Learn by explaining your role to another, and learn to be the patient. Your confidence and abilities will grow with the insights you see flash at you from the other end of the camera.
3. *Always review your work.* Learn from your mistakes. They will teach you more than books and lectures ever will. Take pride in your accomplishments. Ask the doctor to explain your pictures to you. Learn from your efforts. Practice will always improve your work.

Specialized cameras, modelled on the principle of the indirect ophthalmoscope are used to photograph the inner structures of the human eye. Their widespread use in ophthalmology suggests the general medical technician will benefit from the knowledge of basic anatomy and operation of such a camera to take retinal photographs. The technique is easily mastered, if the step-by-step procedure outlined in this chapter is followed.

CHAPTER 6

Stereo Fundus Photography

by J. Michael Coppinger

Binocular stereo vision gives a direct knowledge of the third dimension. Aside from the visual optics involved, stereo is all in the brain's perception. With our two eyes separated horizontally, each eye views an object in space from a slightly different point of view. This separation of the eyes is called the pupillary distance (from the center of one pupil to the center of the other). Using two types of cues, psychological and physiological, each eye sends its separate and slightly different image to the visual cortex for mixing and interpretating as three dimensional sight. A stereo camera duplicates all the circumstances of stereo vision, producing two disparate images, which when viewed in register, reintroduce the third dimension.

Seeing In Stereo

Both the actions of eye and brain, physical cues, and the interpretation of these signals, psychological cues, are necessary to see in three dimensions.

The physiological cues of stereo vision are accommodation and convergence. Accommodation is the adjustment by the eye for seeing at different distances. The crystalline lens changes shape to focus at different distances by the action of the ciliary muscle. Accommodation range decreases with age. Accommodation is only effective when actual or apparent viewing distance is approximately 20 feet or less. Working in combination with accommodation is convergence, the directing of the visual axes of the two eyes to a near point. Muscular tension is necessary to fuse both eye's image(s). Convergence influences accommodation as the visual axes shift from parallel at infinity to sharp convergence at the near point of focus. The lens changes shape as the axes converge. Convergence is ineffective beyond 10 meters, as the visual axes are parallel. The psychological cues of stereo vision are:

- Image size—closer objects appear larger
- Linear perspective—parallel lines converge as they move farther away from the observer

- Shades and shadows and relative position of objects in relation to one another
- Overlapping of surfaces
- Aerial perspective
- Texture gradients

These cues are learned by experience: by the time we can walk and talk we psychologically know these cues.

Simultaneous/Sequential Stereo Photography

In photograph we can duplicate this visual function either simultaneously, using a camera with two separate lenses to record two images *simultaneously;* or we can take a picture with a monocular camera, then shift laterally and take a second image *sequentially.* Both methods work, but only simultaneous photography approximates human vision and produces repeatable photographs with equal stereo separation. Most ophthalmic camera systems are monocular and only sequential stereo photography can be performed. Simultaneous stereo camera systems are available, but infrequently used in clinical practice.

Simultaneous Stereo

In 1957, Dr. David Donaldson introduced two simultaneous stereo camera systems, one for external eye photography and one for fundus photography. These cameras took pairs of images at the same time. Dr. Donaldson's camera used one front objective to create an image. He placed two camera lenses in the optical path to separate this image. The two images passed through modified prisms to two separate eyepieces. The photographer looked through these eyepieces to see and focus. Ironically, because of the number and the position of the camera's prisms and mirrors, the image viewed was reverse stereo, for example, a patient with glaucoma had an optic cup rising up into the vitreous. The film advance system required to record two separate images at the same time on the same roll of film also caused problems. The film was advanced in a two part sequence. First frames 1 and 3 were exposed; then the film advanced one frame only to next expose frames 2 and 4. Then all four frames were moved forward at the same time to allow the next two pairs to be exposed. The film had to be developed and returned uncut so the slides could be correctly paired and mounted. These problems prevented widespread adoption and use of this unique system.

The Zeiss photo slit lamp, using beam splitters and two 35mm camera backs, can record simultaneous stereo images.

Topcon manufactures a camera that produces two images on one 35mm frame of film, called a split frame stereo camera. A special viewer is necessary to view these images.

Sequential stereo retinal photography, that is, taking one then another image, is the usual method taught to ophthalmic photographers. Compare sequential photography to using one eye to see, and constantly moving this eye from the left orbit to the right orbit to create the base separation necessary for depth perception.

Sequential Stereo Photography

Conventional stereo retinal photography is done sequentially by first taking an image then moving the camera sideways to take the second image. The wider the separation of the two images taken, (i.e., the stereo base) the greater the effect of creating three dimensions will be. The eye is a small structure (average axial length 23mm). The stereo base formula is 1 unit sideways for each 30 units of distance from the observation point. The correct stereo base, to accurately represent the depth of tissues involved, would be .75mm. Such a small shift creates accurate but minimally perceptible stereo. To separate the retinal layers for viewing and interpretation, it is necessary to use a larger than normal stereo base, that is, to move laterally farther than .75mm. Such an exaggerated shift produces a conditon called hyper stereo (too much). All retinal photography is hyperstereo, unless the lateral shift is too small.

The performance of sequential stereo photography with a variable angle camera can be very difficult. Variable angle fundus cameras, that is, those equipped with wide angle, standard, and high magnification fields of view require greater dilation of the patient for moncular fundus photography. The wider illumination donut provides less room to shift laterally, within the dilated pupil, consequently the right or left side image may be unevenly illuminated. Accept this limitation and use the brain's power to fuse images to evaluate such stereo pairs.

The manual shift involved in sequential stereo is subjective relative to individual patient dilation, therefore only grossly repeatable. The stereo base of sequential photographs can vary from one pair of images to the next in the same patient. Only simultaneous stereo gives a repeatable and accurate comparable result.

Stereo photography provides useful interpretable information, such as the depth of different changes in the retina, acts as a good teaching tool, and is dramatic and beautiful (the author is a stereo photo addict).

Photographic Method for Stereo Photography

To facilitate stereo fundus photography, maximal dilation is required. A large pupil is necessary to allow lateral shift. The technique for performing sequential stereo photos is simple and easily learned. First align the fundus camera as you would to take a normal photograph. (Figure 6.1). For stereo

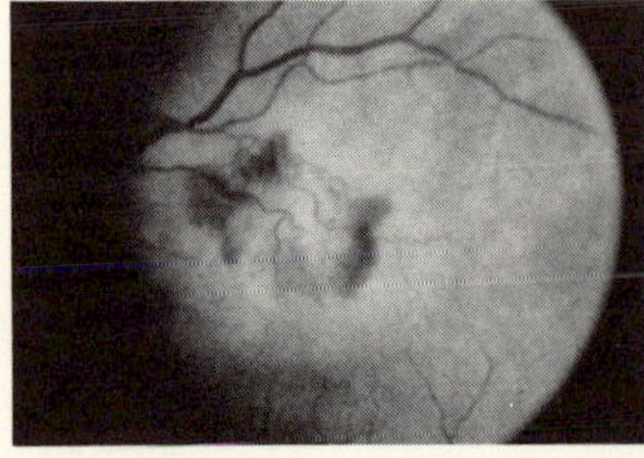

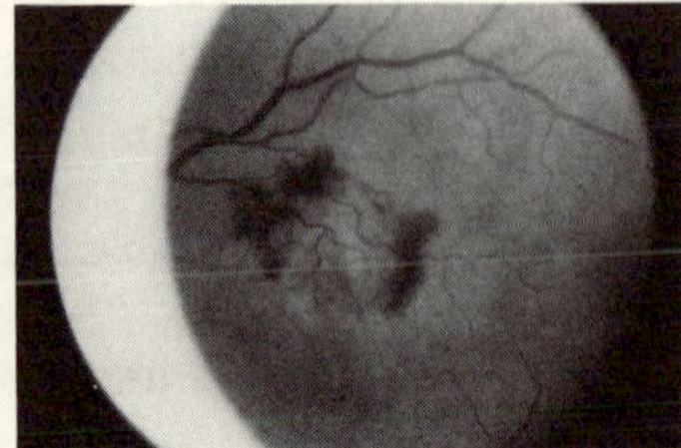

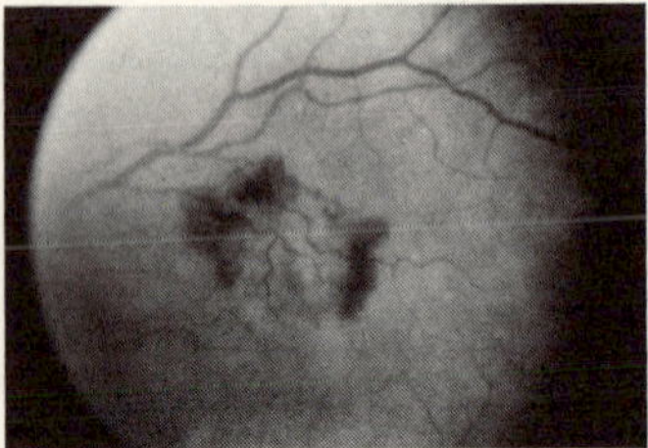

Figure 6.1 A photographic representation of the shift from the center axis (right), through the crescent (center), to the dimmer side image (left). The shift here is from center to the photographer's left. Shifting to the opposite side will also work effectively.

fundus photos, focus on the retina in the center of the pupil. Camera movement is done by moving the joystick or the entire camera base side-to-side, keeping the camera orientation parallel. Move to the right until the yellow crescent appears then *continue* to the right until the reflex minimizes or disappears (Figure 6.1). You will see a dimmer yet useful fundus image. Refocus and take a picture. Next shift back to the left, through the crescent again to the central image, refocus, and shoot a second photo of the stereo pair.

If, when shifting to the right the crescent fails to disappear, pull the camera back toward you slightly to remove it. This same technique can also be accomplished by moving first to the left, then back to the center image. Refer to visualize this pairing. Remember to focus *each* image (Figure 6.2). Preview the stereo pair by moving the camera back and forth before taking an image to ensure you have proper alignment. The side image is dimmer because part of the illumination/light beam falls outside the pupil margin in this position.

Some authors of books on ophthalmic photography describe a method of pairing the left side image with the right side image to create stereo pairs, ignoring the central image in the pairing process. This creates greater hyperstereo than the method above, and ignores the most sharp and useful image the fundus camera can create. Try both methods and compare the results. Both types of sequential stereo photography involve the principle of using corneal induced parallax to take such stereo images. Simply put, the method described by the author works most effectively, especially when doing stereo angiography. A consistent repeatable method is of greatest importance with either technique.

Two stereo pairs are shown in Figure 6.3. The first shows a patient with glaucoma. The optic disc has a cave-like depression centrally. Figure 6.3 shows a patient with an anteriorly swollen optic nerve. In stereo, this pair of images will look like a volcano viewed from above, that is, rising toward the observer. Both pairs of images can be seen in stereo if you view them wearing a trial frame fit with two + 10 lenses.

The patient must maintain fixation to ensure proper stereo sequencing. Stress to the patient you plan to take two pictures in sequence. Ask the patient to hold as still as possible, and if the patient blinks, to return immediately to the fixation target for the second photograph. If the patient moves, begin again. Take a few monocular photographs first to acclimate the patient to the camera flash. Use the crosshairs or reticule as a reference point to insure that the patient is not changing fixation. For example, center the optic disc in the crosshairs (refer to Figure 6.6). Be sure the disc stays in this position for each photo in the pair. The disc will

Patient's direction of gaze:

Directly forward

L, C, and R Represent Illumination Donut in 3 Positions

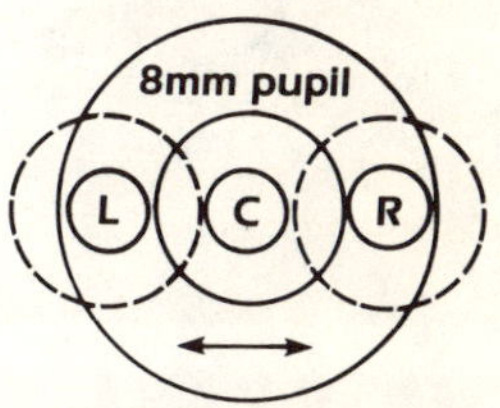

Circular pupil shift (patient looking directly into camera): All pairings must include C image

Figure 6.2a Stereo shift sequence. C must be paired with L or R (top). If you pair L and R, the stereo effect will be greater.

Patient's direction of gaze:
(1) Directly up or down
(2) Directly sideways
(3) Up and in (= down and out)
(4) Up and out (= down and in)

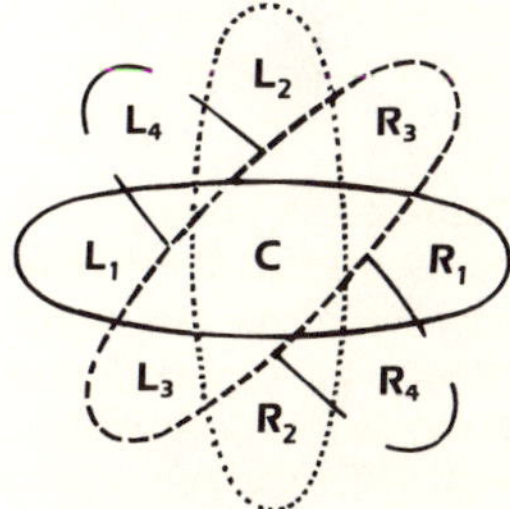

Elliptical pupil shift: All pairings should include C image

Figure 6.2b Stereo shifting across various meridians when the patient's fixation is not straight ahead. Example is for left eye.

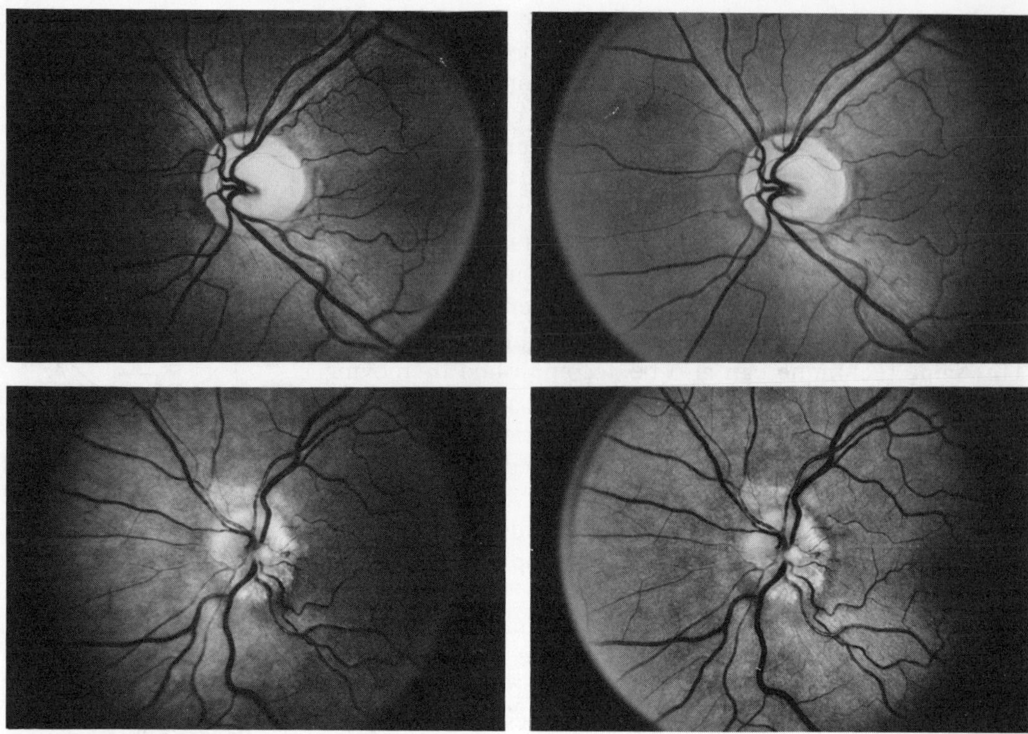

Figure 6.3 A stereo pair of a glaucoma patient (top). A stereo pair of a swollen elevated optic nerve head (bottom). Note the difference in detail focus and illumination in each side of the stereo pair.

move slightly sideways in the eyepiece when you shift side to side.

When photographing the optic disc or macula, the patient's pupil will present a round circle within which a side-to-side shift is readily accomplished. When you photograph the periphery, however the pupil will become oblong, with the widest axis (diameter) perpendicular to the direction of gaze. Shifting should be done across this widest diameter. Temporal or nasal fields may have to be photographed with a vertical rather than horizontal lateral shift (Figure 6.2). Fixation off the horizontal or vertical axis will require both a sideways and an up and down shift to create a good stereo base (Fig. 6.2b) due to elliptical pupil opening.

Stereo Photography of Poorly Dilated Eyes

Small pupils are a deterrant to stereo photos. Although refocusing is urged, when a stereo pair is viewed, only one image need be in sharp focus to fuse the two photos and to see good detail. The second image can be dark or dim. Accept the limits imposed. Take two pictures. Review the photos when the film is processed and see how the stereo images jump out. Such pictures, while hardly ideal, serve the ophthalmologist's needs to help evaluate the patient's eye.

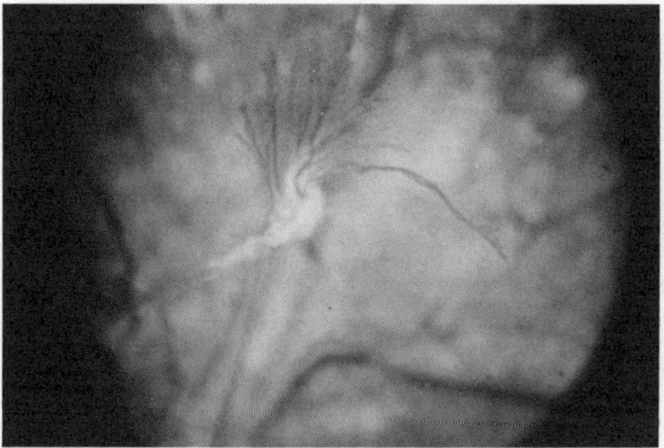

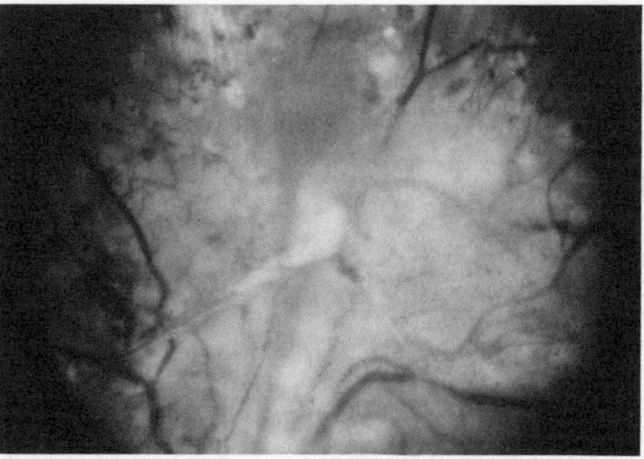

Figure 6.4 Differential focus. This image is focused on the elevated blood vessels in the patient's vitreous (left). After a lateral shift, this image is focused down onto the normal retinal surface (right). When paired, both planes are seen in focus.

Differential Focus

Another technique useful for elevated pathologies is called differential focus. With differential focus, the two pictures taken are each separately focused. One photo, for example the left image, is focused on the retinal blood vessels. After properly shifting laterally, the second photo, the right side of the stereo pair, is refocused at a different level, say, deeper into the area of optic cupping, or with elevated pathologies, in the posterior vitreous. When these two images, focused at different levels, are paired and viewed, your eyes see what they could not otherwise see, two pair planes of focus in the same image in three dimensions (Figure 6.4).

Stereo Viewing Devices

To view stereo pairs you need a stereo viewer. Many types exist. The simplest is to take two 8× optical magnifying loupes, wrap a coat hanger around them and lay one loup over each image. Shift the loupes to adjust for your PD; Use rubber bands to hold them in place. More sophisticated

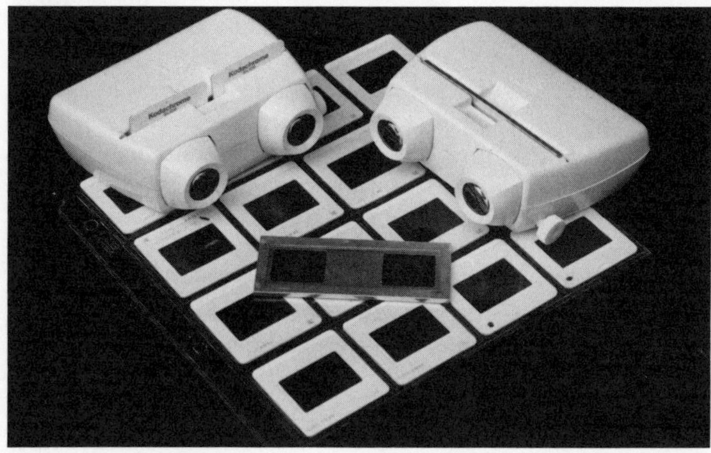

Figure 6.5 One example of a stereo viewer with its own light source. Such viewers work with conventional cardboard slide mounts, as well as special aluminum stereo mounts.

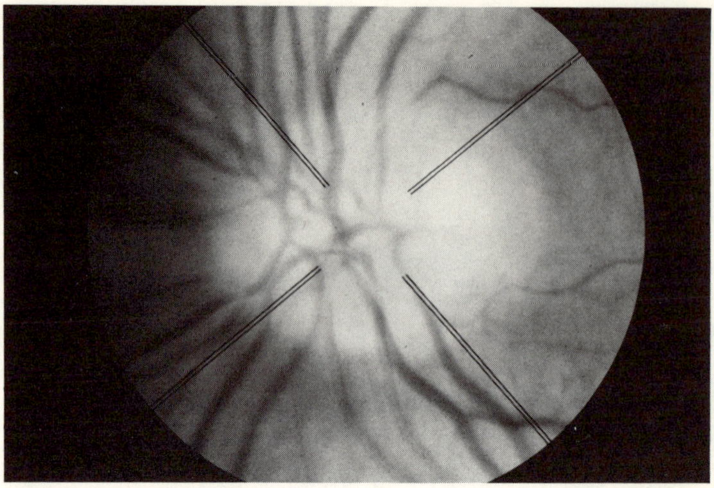

Figure 6.6 This double image with an overlying reticle pattern illustrates two points. One, use the reticle to align the subject, and insure centration from the first image to the second. Two, note the slight change in position of the vessels caused by the lateral shift in making the stereo pair.

viewers can incorporate two similar lenses, a slot for inserting the two slides, a device for adjusting PD, a backlight for transillumination, and a focusing mechanism (Figure 6.5). Another viewer available in all ophthalmologists offices is a trial frame for glasses. Place two (+) 10 diopter lenses in the frame, and view the slides on a light box. For proper viewing, the two slides must be at right angles to the viewer's line of right angles to the viewer's line of vision. The left image must be presented to the left eye, the right image to the right eye.

Tips for stereo fundus photography:

- Use the crosshairs to align each image.
- Do not swing the camera, only shift laterally.
- Use differential focus on all stereo pairs. The patient's lens affects focus, being thicker centrally, thinner peripherally.

Always label slides to indicate which is the left and which is the right image of a stereo pair. Reversing the slides will reverse the stereo effect.

Testing for Stereo Separation

To test for stereo separation, place one slide in its mount over the other and square the corners of the slide mounts. Hold the slides up to a strong light. If one clear overlapped image appears there is no stereo separation. A properly separated pair should present a double image, that is, the same major veins will appear in register approximately 2–3mm apart (Figure 6.6). This indicates a stereo shift has been achieved. Slide the top slide sideways until one overlapped image appears. Note the difference at the edge of the slide mounts. The top slide should be approximately 2 millimeters to the right or left of the one beneath when the images on the slides overlay. The distance necessary to produce an overlap indicates the effective stereo base.

Always test your stereo pairs for base separation using the ovelapping images test.

Applying Stereo to Angiography

Taking the right image first is a useful habit to develop, for when you attempt stereo angiographic images, the sequence

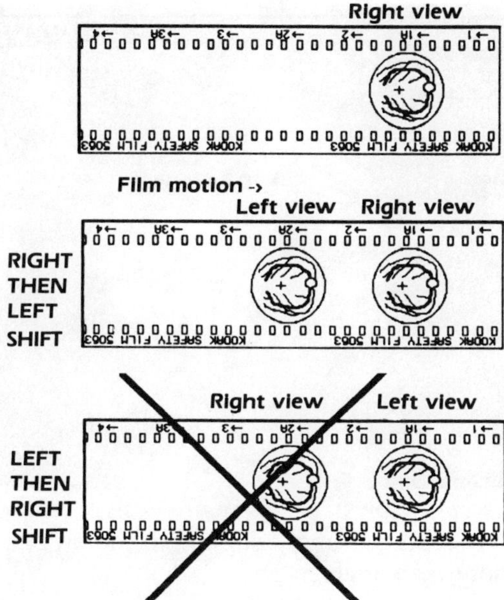

Figure 6.7 Proper sequencing for stereo angiography. Because the film moves from left to right in the camera, the right image must be taken first to present the correct image to the correct eye for viewing. Incorrect shift reverses the stereoscopic effect. (courtesy of Terry King)

of right, then left is *all important*. Figure 6.7 shows two examples of sequencing. Because the film moves through the camera from left to right continuously, any pair to be viewed must present the right image to the right eye, and the left image to the left eye. Taking the left image in a pair first will reverse the stereo effect. The only remedy for this error is to cut the film, and after reversing the images, tape the film together in the correct orientation. Develop the right to left habit while doing fundus photos to facilitate the transition to stereo angiography.

When performing stereo angiographic photos focus only on the center image. If the side image is slightly out of focus, the brain will fuse the focused and nonfocused images after the fact.

Summary

Step-by-step stereo fundus photography

1. Ensure maximum dilation.
2. Focus in the center of the patient's pupil.
3. Move to the left (or right) until the yellow crescent appears; continue to the left (or right) until the reflex disappears or minimizes.
4. Refocus the image.
5. Shoot the photo.
6. Move back to the center image.
7. Refocus and shoot the second image.
   Carefully label slides left and right for later viewing by yourself and the physician when sorting and labeling slides. Review your work and learn more about the eye by seeing the third dimension.

CHAPTER 7

Fluorescein Angiography

by J. Michael Coppinger

All of the principles of camera design and fundus photography technique apply directly to the process of performing fluorescein angiography.

The basic principle of fluorescence depends on a light sensitive material's ability to absorb short wavelengths in the visible spectrum when stimulated, then emit this energy as longer wavelengths when the stimulus is withdrawn.

Fluorescein angiography is the technique of injecting a yellowish dye into a patient's anticubital vein, then photographically stimulating this dye with a blue-green light of certain wavelengths to induce fluorescence in the retinal vascular system of the human eye, and recording this fluorescence on photographic film, using a fundus camera. Unlike fundus photography, which is purely documentary, fluorescein angiography is a diagnostic test yielding information about the patient's ocular health otherwise unavailable to the ophthalmologist. Figure 7.1 is an example of a fluorescein angiogram, a sequential photographic record of this process.

This chapter will focus one the principles, development, and practical techniques involved in fluorescein angiography.

Fluorescence is a property of certain substances, which upon exposure to light of short wavelengths (blue), emits light of longer wavelengths (green-yellow). The dye used in angiography, **sodium fluorescein,** was first synthesized by Von Baeyer in 1871. Dr. Erlich in 1881 injected fluorescein intravenously to study the production of aqueous humor in patients with glaucoma. In 1954, Dr. Maumanee used intravenous fluorescein to study a choroidal hemangioma. He used a cobalt blue filter on a slit lamp to stimulate the dye fluorescence. He did not take photographs, but only observed the injected dye to study ocular tumors. In 1961, Dr. Harold Novotny, a senior medical student, and Dr. David Alvis, an intern, both at Indiana University, began a summer project to study the differences in oxygenation levels in blood vessels for their professor, Dr. John Hickam. Drs. Novotny and Alvis chose the human retina for their subject, because blood

Intravenous fluorescein retinal angiographic photography was developed in 1961 by Drs. Harold Novotny and David Alvis.

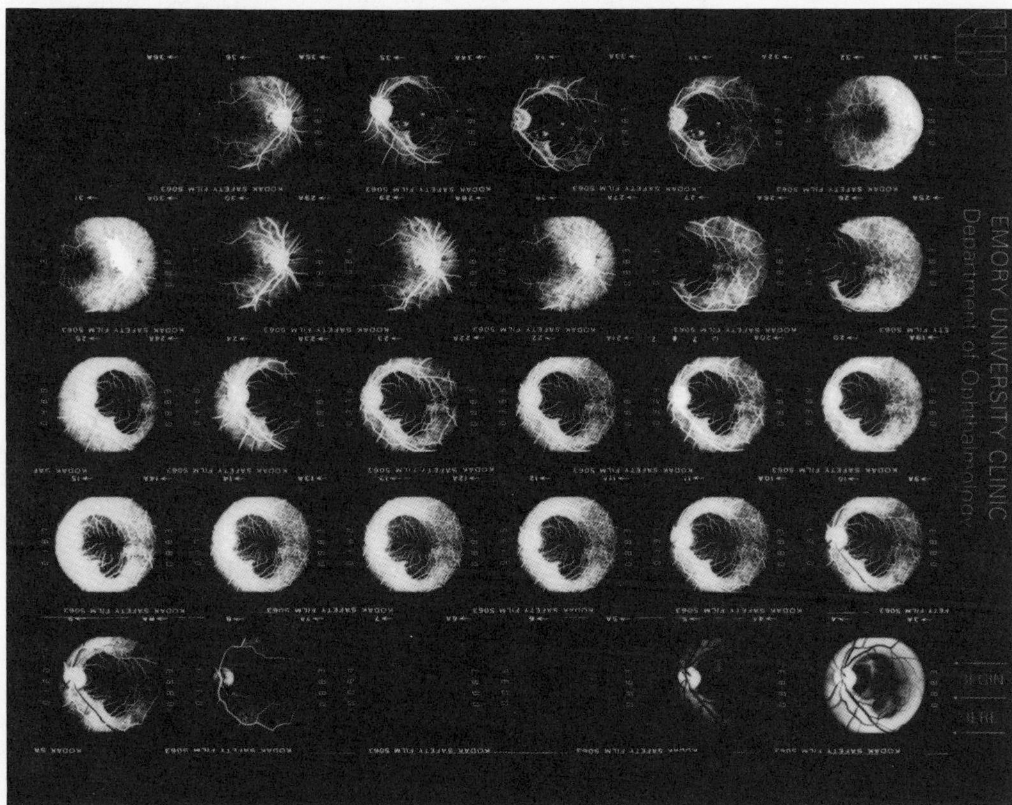

Figure 7.1 A contact positive of a fluorescein angiogram. Sequence begins at the lower left image and follows to upper right. Times at the left of each image are postdye injection (in seconds). The contact print is oriented with the frame numbers upside down, because a fundus camera inverts the image twice instead of once as in a conventional 35 mm camera.

vessels were easily seen using a Zeiss fundus camera in their lab. As Dr. Novotny worked with the fundus camera an idea took shape in his mind. If he could find an injectable material which would, when injected into a patient's blood system, fluoresce, the aims of his summer job might be greatly expanded, and "we might do some very interesting things."

Pursuing this idea, Dr. Novotny received permission to remove the side of the camera and look inside. To achieve fluorescence, Dr. Novotny placed various filters in a revolving disc between the flash tube/view lamp position and the objective lens of the camera, so the light entering the patient's eye was of only particular wavelengths. Realizing that only the fluorescence induced must reach the camera after exiting the patient's eye, he then placed a barrier filter in the mouth of the 35mm camera body. This filter (green) blocked the stimulating light (blue) from reaching the film (hence barrier) and permitted only the actual fluorescence to pass through and be recorded on the camera's film. Dr. Novotny worked with the Eli-Lilly pharmaceutical house in Indianapolis to perfect the dye to be used, eventually arriving at sodium fluorescein as his intravenous dye. He was unaware that others were already using fluorescein. He then experimented with various films and developers to find the best combination of materials to record this fluorescent dye transit.

Drs. Novotny and Alvis began by photographing rabbits. Then, finding their method worked, Dr. Novotny attempted the first human retinal angiogram on Dr. David Alvis. He succeeded in recording the details of the dye transit on film. Limiting factors caused problems. Flash recycling time (the speed at which pictures could be taken sequentially) was very slow. Dr. Alvis could only take one picture each 12 seconds. Subsequent replacement of the exposure tube with a high powered electronic flash allowed more rapid recording of the dye filling sequence. (Today some fundus cameras take as many as 3 pictures per second.)

Drs. Novotny and Alvis wrote a paper describing their findings and submitted it to the *American Journal of-phthalmology*. The editor of the AJO rejected the paper as unoriginal work. Drs. Novotny and Alvis then published the paper in the *Archives of Circulation*—a cardiology journal. As of this writing, 26 years later, though fundus cameras and filters have been improved, the technique developed by these two men remains the same and is in use around the world every day.

Prominent ophthalmologists read the article and recognized the significance of this new technique. Dr. Novotny went on to become a psychiatrist, but the diagnostic tool he developed literally rewrote the textbooks on retinal and choroidal disease.

Fluorescein Dye and Its Characteristics

In chemical terms, sodium fluorescein is a compound of carbon$_{20}$, hydrogen$_{10}$, sodium$_{2}$, and oxygen$_{5}$. When reacting with sodium hydroxide it forms a stable sodium salt. It is compounded as a fluorescein acid-free equivalent. In powdered form, fluorescein is an orange-red crystalline hydrocarbon. Mixed in a dilute alkaline solution it becomes yellow with green fluorescence. The absorbtion peak is 465–490 nanometers (blue).The emission peak is 520–530 nanometers (green).

Injectable fluorescein will not emit fluorescence unless bound with another solution. When injected into the body, the dye binds with serum protein in the blood. In this bound state the dye will fluoresce with blue light radiation when excited. This physical reaction occurs as the fluorescein absorbs the blue light. The added electrons elevate fluorescein to a higher energy state. As with other excited molecules, when the stimulus is withdrawn, the fluorescein molecule has a tendency to return to its ground state. Fluorescein molecules do this by emitting a characteristic yellow-greenish light that is the light recorded as fluorescence. Fluorescein exhibits specific physical properties that are necessary to know. Maximum fluorescence occurs at PH 7.4. When bound to the albumen in serum protein there is a reduction in fluorescence by conjunction with adjacent hemoglobin molecules. There is no firm bond with vital tissues. Fluorescein rapidly diffuses through intracellular and extracellular spaces. Fluorescein is eliminated through the kidneys and liver within 24 to 48 hours.

An understanding of the physical properties of sodium resorcenol (commonly called fluorescein) is required for the certification of a photographer. This author recommends all photographers have a fluorescein angiogram to experience life in front of the camera instead of behind it. When a photographer tells a patient "I've had this test and I'm still alive" the resulting laugh breaks the tension, and relieves the fear the patient is experiencing.

Fluorescein stains skin and mucous membranes for 2 to 4 hours. Fluorescein causes yellow-orange discoloration of the urine for 1 to 2 days, which creates false positive results in urine tests for reducing sugar levels. Fluorescein diffuses freely in the eye through the choriocapillaris, Bruch's membrane, the sclera, and portions of the optic nerve, but not through retinal pigment epithelium, the retinal blood vessels or large choroidal vessels. This normal diffusion pattern is the key to fluorescein angiographic interpretation (more later on this subject).

Major indications for retinal fluorescein angiography are:

- retinal pigment epithelial abnormalities
- choroidal exudative diseases
- retinal vascular diseases
- differential for macular/optic nerve diseases
- differential diagnosis of intraocular tumors, and
- malingering.

Physical Reactions to Fluorescein

Contraindications for retinal fluorescein angiography are:

- Pregnancy—don't be shy; ask any woman in her childbearing years if she is or may be pregnant. No adverse results have been reported, yet here it is wise to err on the side of caution.
- A previous history of reaction,
- Where diagnosis and treatment are obvious,
- The patient with a history of multiple allergies.

There are two categories of reactions, minor and major. Minor reactions reported are sneezing, tongue parasthesia, local pain at the injection site due to dye infiltration, nausea and vomiting (approximately 2% of patients), dizziness, pruritis (itching) and uticaria (hives).

Potential patient reactions to fluorescein dye, while relatively uncommon, can occur. Protect the patient and yourself by knowing the signs of specific reactions. Have the medical supplies on hand to manage such reactions, and know how to use them. Get CPR certified. Never perform angiograms without a physician *in the office* and available to manage a fluorescein dye reaction.

Major reactions reported are syncope (swooning or fainting), allergic respiratory reaction (loss of breath), hypertension, shock, cardiac failure, basilar artery ischemia, and pulmonary edema. Serious reactions are rare.

As with any invasive procedure, certain precautions should always be taken to ensure the ability to deal with any of these reactions. Most of the reactions listed are rare, but you must be ready for any of them. An emergency kit and oxygen should always be at hand when performing angiography. Keep all medications current. Replace outdated supplies in your emergency kit regularly.

Treatments for Adverse Reactions

Nausea is usually transitory, occuring after full venous filling. Have the patient sit back. Ask the patient to breathe deeply and evenly in for a count of four, hold the breath for one second, then breathe out to a count of four. This technique of yoga breathing will usually relieve the discomfort, and avoid the need for the emesis basin or bucket. If there is a history of a previous reaction of this type, you can administer oral phenergan (25—50mg.) one hour prior to performing the test.

Fainting is best handled with smelling salts. Monitor the blood pressure and pulse for an appropriate interval. Administer oxygen, if necessary. Place the patient in a supine position as soon as possible, and raise his or her feet.

Infiltration of dye at the injection site is extremely painful for the patient. An ice pack will relieve the discomfort. Administration of aspirin or acetominophen may also be desirable for the duration of the pain. In a severe case, a subcutaneous injection of lidocaine will relieve the pain quickly.

Hives and other allergic reactions should be treated with oral or intravenous Benadryl.

Bronchospasm or anaphylaxis should be treated as a life threatening situation. Open the airway immediately. Oxygenate the patient. Call Code Blue/the doctor. Yes, this is serious. Your emergency kit (imperative to have on hand) should contain an intravenous pack, oral airway tube, a stethascope, oxygen, a sphygmomanometer (an instrument for measuring the tension of blood current or arterial pressure), a portable hand resuscitator, sterile needles, syringes, tube connectors, as well as the following systemic medications (current): steroids (IV Solucortef), antihistamines (oral and IV), epinephrine (subcutaneous), aminophylline (IV), pressor agents, bicarbonate, lidocaine, and benadryl. Also make sure you have an emesis basin, an ice pack, and an area to lay the patient supine. CPR training for the photographer should be mandatory in all situations. Know how to use all the supplies in your emergency kit. If you don't, have your doctor teach you.

While many of these reactions are uncommon, they might happen to you. Be prepared to assist the doctor.

Administration of Fluorescein

Fluorescein has many other applications in medicine. Dermatologists use it to study the skin. Radiologists use it to study internal vasculature in combination with radioactive isotopes using x-rays.

Fluorescein is applied by ophthalmologists to topically stain the cornea. Intravenous injection is done to study iris, aqueous, ciliary process and conjunctivae, as well as vitreous and retina.

Other dyes are also used to study the fundus. Among them are indocyanine, pyranine, rhodamine, and NK-1841. Some of these dyes pass quicky through the system and dissipate. None of these dyes is used in conventional retinal angiography, but instead for research and experimentation.

Fluorescein is usually administered intravenously in the anticubital vein through a loaded syringe and butterfly infusion needle. A saline flush is sometimes injected following fluorescein to push the dye bolus through the butterfly tubing and into the patient's vein. The saline can also be injected prior to the dye to ensure infiltration does not occur when in doubt about the vein's integrity or the position of the butterfly needle.

Oral administration of fluorescein was first done in 1910 by Dr. Burke. He administered 5 grams of dye mixed with coffee to adults (less for children) and observed their fundus in white light. This oral technique works effectively. Mix a vial of dye with soda or vegetable juice. Have the patient drink it. Delivery time to the eye is approximately 15 to 20 minutes. Use a higher than normal flash setting on the camera to record the image. Filling is diffuse and cumulative, rather than sudden as in the intravenous bolus method. Maximum fluorescence occurs at 20-40 minutes.

Oral fluorescein is not commonly used for photographic studies.

Fluorescein is available in different concentrations. The two most common use are 5cc of 10% solution or 2 or 3cc's of 25% solution. Either dilution works effectively.

Filtration

For angiography, your camera must be equipped with special filters. A blue exciter filter and a yellow-green barrier filter have already described. Before we discuss angiographic technique, let's look at these and the other filters in the camera. Figure 7.2 shows a graph. Measured along the x (horizontal) axis are the wavelengths of light from ultra violet 300 nanometers through blue (400 NM), green (550 NM), to red (700 NM) and finally infrared (800 NM). Vertically we measure % of transmission of light.

The filter equation: Blue light into the eye; green and blue out. The barrier stops the blue; the film records the green.

To take a fundus photograph, we use the entire visible spectrum or white light. This full daylight exposure yields colors as the normal eye sees them. When we perform angiography we use two segments of the spectrum. First we filter the light going into the patient's eye with a bluish filter (465–490 NM). This filter allows only these restricted wavelengths to pass through from the "white light" flashtube in the camera. This blue light strikes the intravenous dye in the eye of the patient and temporarily "excites" the dye to a higher energy state. After each flash, the excited dye loses this energy and emits light of longer wavelengths—green/yellow, (peak at 520–530 NM). Some of the blue light entering the eye is scattered and reflected back out of the eye along with the green light.

Only the green light is true fluorescence, so only this green light should reach the black-and-white film in the camera back. So, a barrier filter which blocks the reflected blue light from reaching the film in a position must be placed so it filters only the light exiting the patient's eye. This filter must be positioned at or near the 35mm camera holding the film. An ideal combination of exciter and barrier filters would have no overlap on the graph. The ideal world is not here yet. Even the best filter sets have a minimal crossover that allows some blue light to reach the film (Figure 7.2).

Dr. Novotny began using filters for angiography that had significant overlap. This overlap allowed much blue light to reach the film. Photographs taken prior to the dye injection recorded detail on the film even though there was no fluorescence. This condition of filter overlap is called pseudo (or fake) fluorescence (Figure 7.3).

This recording of detail prior to injection led many doctors and photographers to look for better combinations of filters

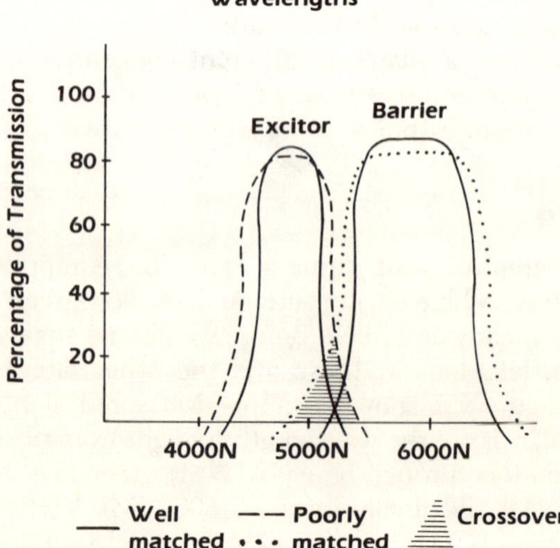

Figure 7.2 Comparison of well matched excitor/barrier filters, and a poorly matched pair. The crossover indicates blue light is reaching the film.

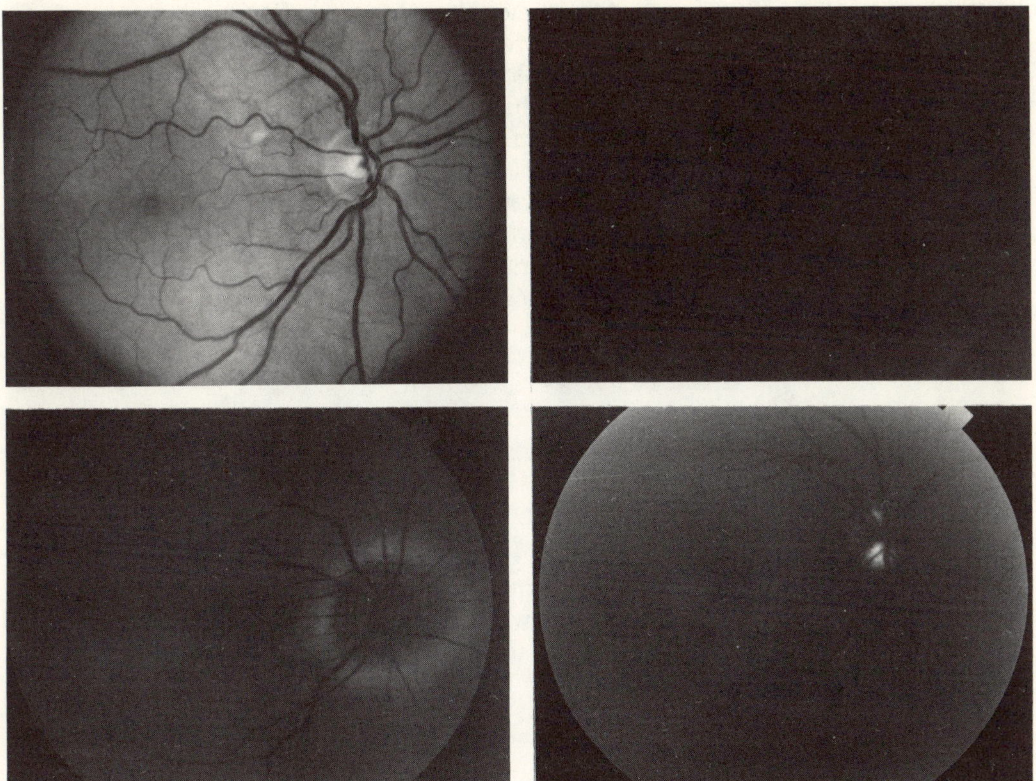

Figure 7.3 "Red Free" photo taken with a green filter prior to introduction of fluorescein filters (top left). Preinjection control photo through well matched filters produces no image (top right). Control photo through poorly matched filters demonstrating pseudofluorescence (bottom left). Autofluorescence from optic nerve head drusen (bottom right).

to eliminate the overlapping pseudofluorescence. Dr. Haining and Roger Lancaster in 1969 designed filters that almost completely eliminated the overlap. Since then Dr. Francois DeLori and Mr. George Zondiros designed a set of filters that produced only 0.1% overlap. These filters are found in many retinal cameras today. Recently the camera manufacturers have begun producing filters for use in their own fundus cameras. Check your for overlap by taking a photograph of each patient prior to the injection. Well matched filters will show no detail on this frame (Figure 7.3).

Some ocular retinal conditions produce their own fluorescence. The most common of these is optic nervehead drusen (Figure 7.3). A photograph taken through even well matched filters prior to dye injection will record detail on the film due to the fluorescent properties of the pathology. This fluorescence is real and called auto (self) fluorescence.

Filters have a life span. They wear out with use or exposure to humidity. The exciter filter will die from edge to center as the layers of gels in the filter separate. If the excitor filter can be removed from your fundus camera, hold it up to a light. The center will be darker with a lighter ring around it if there is wear. This wear can be confirmed with a control photograph taken of the patient prior to injection of fluorescein. If the filters are wearing, detail will be visible on the

Check the filters regularly for wear. If the filters cannot be removed, take a control photo before the dye injection with both filters in position. Check the films after development. Always check the negatives. Look for detail in the control picture. Detail indicates wear (or poor filter matching.)

frame. The barrier filter should also be checked regularly for wear. Some barrier filters can be withdrawn from the fundus camera and held up to the light. Others, mounted in the 35mm camera back, must be inspected after being removed from the camera, or by looking through the camera body at a light with the camera back open. The filter can be examined by firing the camera shutter a few times while looking through the shutter from the film's position. Replace both excitor and barrier filter when the excitor wears excessively. Each pair of fluorescein filters is matched, and replacing only the excitor will still produce some overlap or pseudo-fluorescence.

Fluorescein Angiography: Technique

To maximize performing a fluorescein angiogram, we will divide the technique into 5 parts and treat each one separately. They are as follows: the patient, the set-up, the injection, the photo plan, and the photographer and the doctor.

The Patient

In the explanation of the test, stress the following points:

- The test is photographic, not x-ray.
- The dye is injected into the vein in the arm, ". . . like having blood drawn . . .".
- There are two noticeable side effects: "your skin will turn yellow for approximately two hours." (This is because the dye circulates throughout the entire body.) And, "your urine will be discolored yellow-orange for one to two days" (the dye is eliminated through the kidneys).

Ask for a history of previous allergic reactions. If the patient has reacted to any types of medications, alert the doctor, and proceed only as the doctor advises. Many older patients have had allergic reactions to sulfa and penicillin many years ago; this often does not cause problems. You are looking for *serious* reactions to iodine or other contrast mediums, or previous reaction to fluorescein.

Warn the patient of transient nausea that may follow the injection—this frequently occurs after the initial transit phase. If the patient complains, have the patient sit back, breathe deeply in, hold, and breathe slowly out. Repeat as in Yoga breathing 4 counts in, 1 count hold, 4 counts out. Repeat two or three times. The "wave" effect will generally pass. Have an emesis basin ready if it does not.

Informed Consent

Fluorescein angiography is an invasive procedure with potentially serious side effects. Therefore, informed consent is mandatory. *Written* informed consent is *highly advised* (the redundancy is deliberate). The doctor ordering an angiogram has the responsibility to explain the test to the patient. Even when a doctor explains angiography to a patient, the patient, often in an emotional state, fails to hear or understand the doctor's explanation.

Informed consent should be obtained after a complete explanation to the patient of the test to be performed.

The photographer must reexplain the test to the patient, and obtain written permission on a consent form when so required. A written explanation is most useful in allaying patient fears. This form may vary from a general surgical consent form to a highly detailed form outlining the reasons for and complications of fluorescein angiography. Dilated patients should have the form read to them, so they know what they are signing. The ideal course of action is to: give the patient a written explanation to read; answer any questions the patient may have about the test; explain the informed consent form to the patient and explain possible side effects to the patient; ask the patient to sign the form; dilate the patient. The more attention paid to explaining the test to the patient, the more relaxed and cooperative the patient will *usually* be. Knowledge will often allay the fear of the test the patient may be experiencing. A cooperative patient yields better angiograms.

The Injection Kit

While the patient is dilating, prepare the essential supplies to inject fluorescein: 19-, 21-, 23-gauge butterfly infusion kits (Figure 7.4; various gauge needles are needed for different sized veins); syringes loaded with fluorescein; alcohol wipes; a tourniquet; bandaids; a complete emergency kit (see previous description of "adverse reactions"); micropore tape. Additional recommended supplies are: a syringe loaded with saline; cotton swabs to hold eye lids; arm rest on camera table; a small lamp to illuminate injection site; and filtration aspiration needles with built in filters to draw fluorescein (this catches the small pieces of glass that fall into the fluorescein solution when the glass ampules are broken and the fluorescein drawn through a needle into the syringe). Preloaded syringes avoid this problem, but are more expensive. Fluorescein also comes in rubber topped vials from which the dye is drawn with a conventional needle, as we would a bacteriostatic saline. No glass is broken in this method.

Prepare the necessary supplies for the injection of fluorescein while the patient is still dilating.

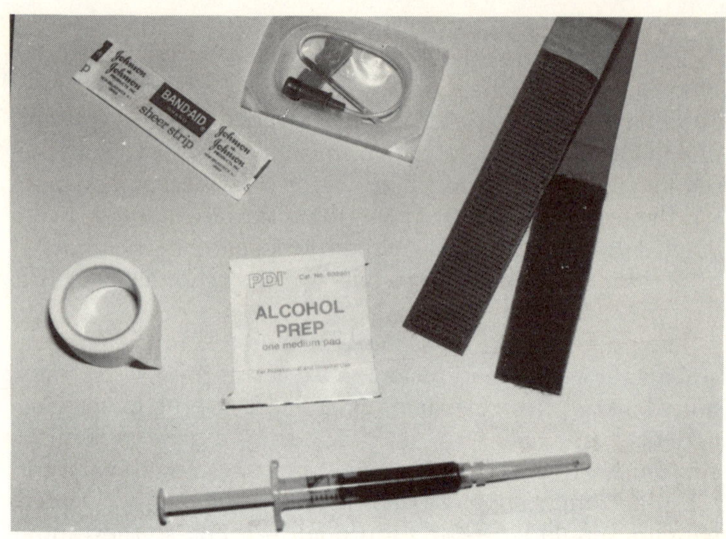

Figure 7.4 The standard kit for I.V. fluorescein injection includes tourniquet, syringe loaded with dye, alcohol, tape, butterfly and bandaid.

The Set-up

Coordination between injector and photography is *the* crucial event during a fluorescein angiogram. When the preliminary steps have been completed (fundus photos, red-free photos, nametag photo, control photos), reassure the patient by re-explaining the basic procedure, as you did with the consent form (Figure 7.3). Then either get someone to inject the dye, or prepare to do it yourself. Whether you do your own injection or have someone else do it while you perform the photography, the following form should be observed (refer to Figure 7.5):

In almost every state in the USA, only Medical Doctors and Registered Nurses may perform any kind of intravenous injection. Know the law in your state.

1. Position the patient at the camera, prior to inserting the needle.
2. Introduce the fixation target and align the camera on the area to be photographed during initial dye transit.
3. Position the patient's arm comfortably.
4. Apply the tourniquet. Use the anticubital vein or the back of the hand (Figure 7.5). Ask the patient which arm has a better vein; patients usually know where blood is successfully drawn.
5. Insert the butterfly needle into the vein (Figure 7.5).
6. Remove the tourniquet.
7. Check the bloodflow by allowing the blood to flow to the syringe. The blood will be injected into the vein first. If the dye is pushed down from syringe to the butterfly needle before the butterfly is inserted into the patient's vein, the first fluid injected is dye, and if infiltration occurs, the level of discomfort for the patient may make further attempts at injection more difficult, and diminish the quality of the test.

A smoothly executed injection will invariably improve the quality of the study being performed. A rushed injection will often negate the value of the test.

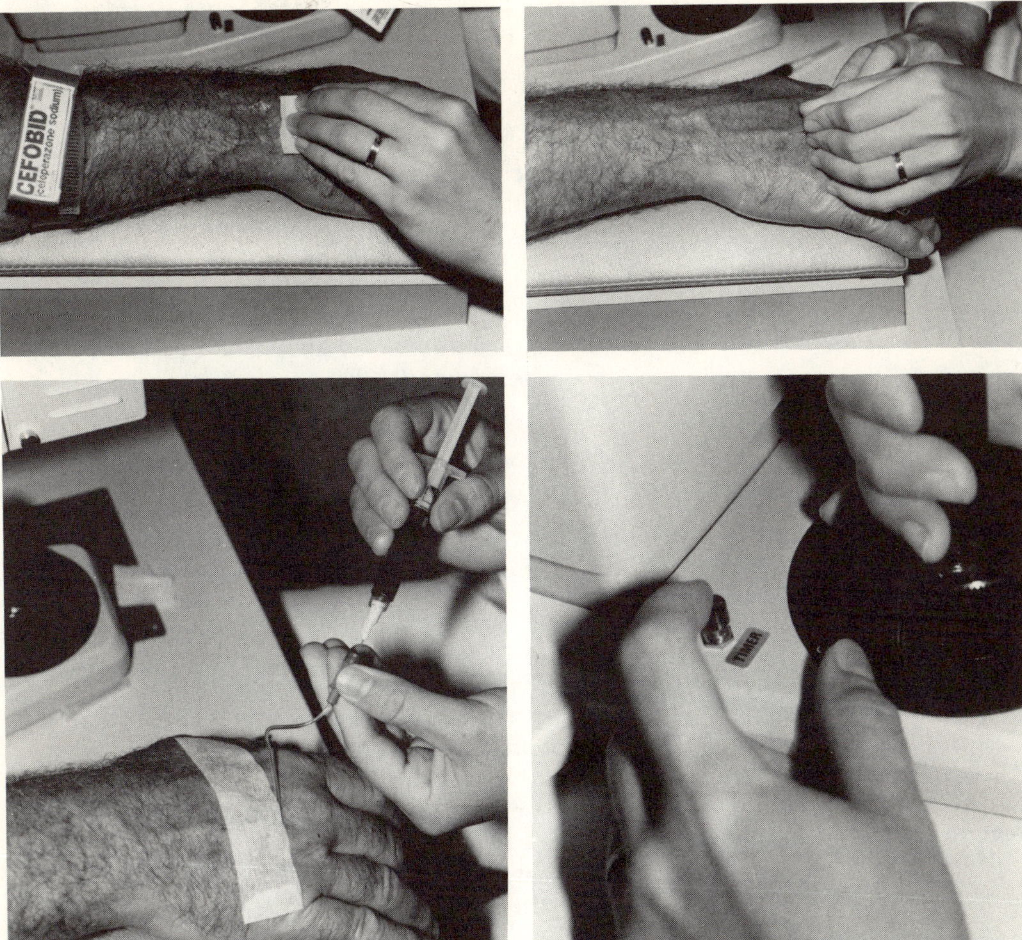

Figure 7.5 Injection technique: Clean the site with alcohol (top left). Insert the butterfly needle. Attach syringe to butterfly—check for blood-flow (top right; bottom left). Start the timer as the injection begins (bottom right).

8. Inform the photographer when ready.
9. The photographer should recheck alignment, and *tell* the injector to "go." Unless the photographer is the controlling agent, the injection may proceed without the photographer's knowledge, and the study can be compromised. The dye moves rapidly to the eye and the dye may pass through arteries and veins before any photos can be taken. This often happens when people are rushed.
10. The photographer should start the timing device on the camera at the "go" signal. The injector should deliver the dye at roughly 1 cc/sec (Figure 7.5).
11. The speed of injection will be determined by the vascular integrity of the patient. However, an injection that takes more than 10–12 seconds is too slow. The dye should appear as a strong bolus in the eye. Dripping the dye into the patient's vein will reduce contrast on the film.
12. A saline flush (5cc) is recommended to push the dye as quickly as possible through the heart to the eye.

13. The injector should wait at least until the initial sequence of photos to remove the IV from the patient's arm. A photographer who performs the injections will need to modify this plan. Beginning to intermediate photographers should depend on someone else for help until they are familiar in the photographic side of the procedure, before taking on the added role of injector.

There are different regulations about who may inject patients in each state. Find out what the rules are before beginning to do your own injections. Always be sure the doctor is in the office when doing IV fluorescein injections.

The Photo Plan

The following list is a step-by-step guide to performing fundus photography in combination with fluorescein angiography. The sequence of events is as follows:

1. Inform the patient as to the nature of the test.
2. Obtain a written consent.
3. Dilate the patient as widely as possible.
4. Allow the patient to sit in the waiting area. Return to the photo room.
5. Turn on the camera system.
6. Check that the camera lens is clean.
7. Load the camera backs with film.
8. Check that the eyepiece crosshairs are focused.
9. Prepare the injection kit.
10. Bring the patient to the photo room.
11. Seat the patient comfortably at the camera.
12. Introduce the fixation device to the patient. Ask the patient to identify what can be seen. This way you can learn the limits of the individual's ability to fixate for the angiogram.
13. Ask the patient to close both eyes.
14. Align the camera, projecting the viewlamp filament (the "donut") on the patient's eyelid, with the joystick in an upright position.
15. Ask the patient to open both eyes.
16. Perform fundus photography, focusing sharply on the center of each image.
17. Let the patient rest when fundus photography is completed.
18. Change camera backs to the one loaded with fluorescein black and white film. Check to see that the film is properly loaded.
19. Photograph a name tag (usually through a green filter at a low flash setting.) Some cameras have a slot to insert a name plate that imprints the patient's name on each photograph. If you use this,

The main points in the angiographic procedures are:

1. Take color fundus photos of both eyes.
2. Make sure the camera is properly loaded with the correct film.
3. Explain the test thoroughly to the patient.
4. Take pictures with a green filter of both eyes prior to the injection.
5. Set up the I.V. for the injection.
6. Reposition the patient.
7. Begin the injection.
8. Start photography 5–10 seconds after the injection begins, slowly at first, then more rapidly until dye arrives in the eye, filling arteries then veins.
9. Photograph the other eye as quickly as possible after full venous filling.
10. Take late photos of both eyes at 7–10 minutes post-injection.

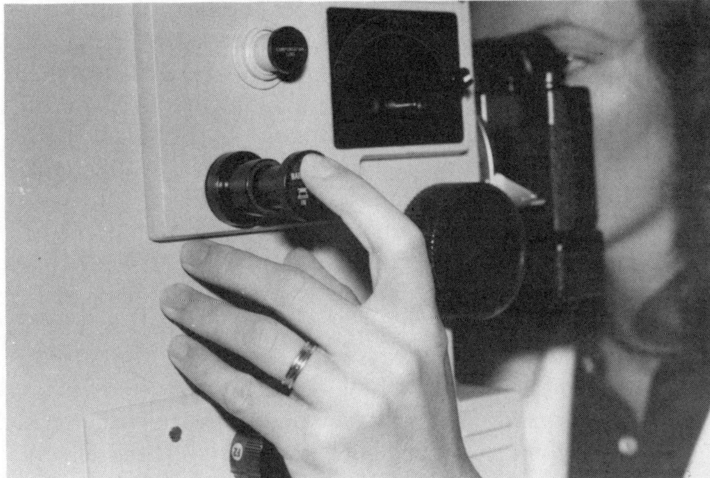

Figure 7.6 The barrier filter in the position where the photographer must look through it to take photographs (left). Inserting/removing the barrier filter to check focus (bottom left). Camera system with a separate eyepiece. Barrier filter is in the 35mm camera below. A light yellow filter can be taped over the eyepiece to enhance contrast (bottom right).

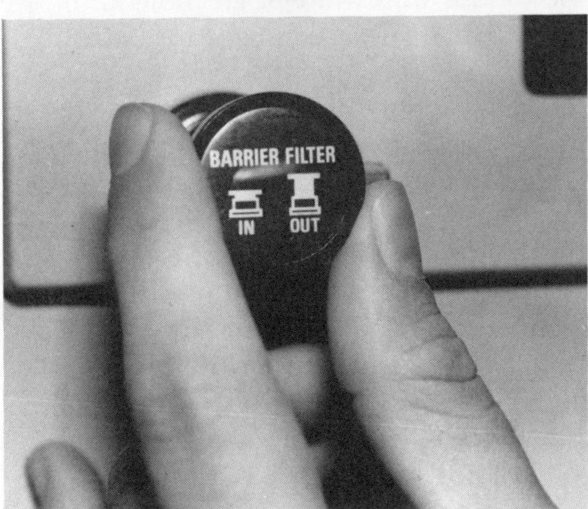

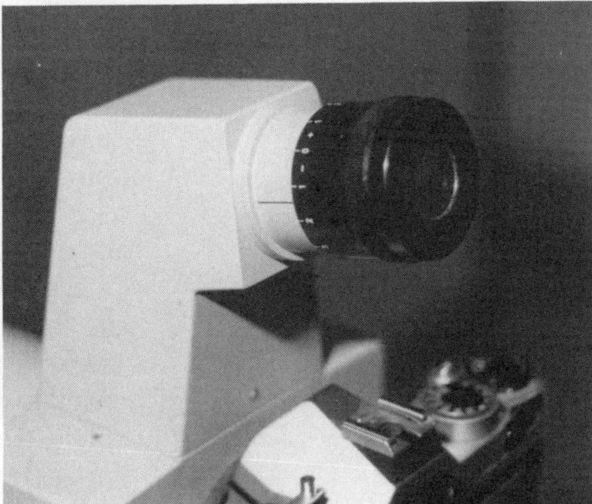

check the correct name is on the tag.

20. Reposition the patient for photography.
21. Take "red-free" photos, using the camera's green filter, of both eyes, concentrating on the area of interest for the fluorescein transit series (e.g,. macula OU). Take a picture of the noninvolved eye first, then the involved eye (the eye in which the dye transit will be photographed).
22. Remove the green filter.
23. Insert the blue exciter filter and confirm the correct field of view for the fluorescein. If your fundus camera does not have a barrier filter in the light path to your eye this is the view you will continue to see prior to dye transit (blue light only). To see fluorescence in blue light only, it is necessary to be dark adapted, or you may not appreciate the dye flowing through the retinal blood vessels. To enhance contrast, put a Wrattan gelatin 12 filter over the eyepiece of the camera (Figure 7.6). This light yellow filter enhances contrast when viewing dye

transit. Its use also eliminates the need for the photographer to dark adapt to see fluorescence.

Many newer fundus cameras have a barrier filter placed between the camera's objective lens and the camera eyepiece mirror (Figure 7.6). This filter must be prior to photographing dye transit or blue light reaches the film. This barrier filter like the 12 Wrattan gel filter, also enhances contrast for the photographer while viewing dye transit. When the barrier filter is between the patient's eye and the photographer's eye, if the filters are well matched, nothing is visible. Only two ways exist to confirm correct position while photographing through the exciter/barrier combination. One is to remove the barrier temporarily, the other, to remove both exciter/and barrier filters and view the fundus with white or green light.

Check patient position by removing the barrier filter, and view the patient's fundus through blue excitor light. Reinsert the barrier filter to take *ALL* pictures of dye.

It is best to prefocus with green light for both patient comfort as well as optimal focus for the pictures. Green-yellow light is the color of the light passing through the barrier filter and reaching the film plane. Due to chromatic abberation, various wavelengths of light are focused at different points of depths in the film. With green light focus those wavelengths of light that will record on the film are as sharply focused as possible. Even newer cameras have a barrier filter that flips in for the picture, then back out for observation. Once dye transit is complete the filter can be left in for viewing and scanning the retina for other pictures.

24. Make certain the power flashing setting is set correctly for fluorescein angiography.
25. Set the timer on the camera to zero. This timer records the dye transit time on the film. As you take serial photographs, the time elapsed since injection is printed beside each picture (Figure 7.3).
26. Allow the patient to rest while you set up the injection kit, and get the doctor or nurse for the injection. Be sure to reassure the patient, reexplain the test if necessary, and emphasize the importance of the dye transit sequence. Tell the patient "The dye will move rapidly into the eye. Try to watch the target. If you blink, open wide again. We'll take about 10–15 pictures in rapid sequence."
27. Proceed with the dye injection and start with this photo plan for the angiogram. Figure 7.7 is a photo plan for the angiogram designed by Sheila Smith-Brewer, of Cleveland, Ohio. It outlines the various common disease entities most commonly requiring fluorescein angiography. This chart concisely defines both sequencing and areas of interest for any par-

AREAS TO DOCUMENT ON FA

* = MOST IMPORTANT PHASE OF FA

DISEASE	EARLY	MID PHASE	VENOUS PHASE	LATES 7-9 MIN.
BDR BACKGROUND DIABETIC RETINOPATHY	30° *Macula/Disc (Look for leaking microaneurysms)	60° 45° 30° Nasal/Temporal Disc/Macula	60° 45° 30° Sweep Periphery Shot of Iris O.U.	30° *Macula/Disc (Stereo) (Document CME)
PRE PDR PRE-PROLIFERATIVE DIABETIC RETINOPATHY	30° *Macula/Disc	60° 45° 30° Nasal/Temporal Disc/Macula	60° 45° 30° Sweep Periphery (Document areas of capillary non-perfusion) (Document areas of NVE vs. IRMA) Shot of Iris O.U.	30° Macula/Disc (Stereo)
PDR PROLIFERATIVE DIABETIC RETINOPATHY	60° 45° 30° Macula/Disc (Document NVD)	60° 45° 30° Nasal/Temporal Disc/Macula	60° 45° 30° *Sweep Periphery (Document NVE) (Document areas of capillary non-perfusion) Shot of Iris O.U. (Document Rubeosis — leakage at pupillary margin)	60° 45° 30° Macula/Disc (Stereo)
SMCD SENILE MACULAR CHOROIDAL DEGENERATION	30° Only *Macula (Disc, if parapapillary) (look for CNV) Early Leakage (Clear FAZ important)	30° Macula/Disc	30° 20° Macula Scan Periphery	30° Only *Macula (10-15 min. lates) (Look for increased hyperfluorescence)
CME CYSTOID MACULAR EDEMA IRVINE GASS SYNDROME	30° Macula/Disc	30° Macula/Disc	30° Macula/Disc Scan Periphery	15-20 Min. 30° *Macula/Disc (Look for flower-petal pooling pattern) (Document hyperfluorescent disc) (Stereo)
CRVO CENTRAL RETINAL VEIN OCCLUSION	60° 45° 30° Disc	60° 45° 30° Disc/Macula	60° 45° 30° *Sweep Periphery (Document areas of capillary non-perfusion) (Differentiate collateral vessels from NVD) Shots of Iris (Document Rubeosis)	60° 45° 30° Disc/Macula (Look for Macular Edema — CME)
BVO BRANCH VEIN OCCLUSION	60° 45° 30° Macula/and Affected Quadrant	60° 45° 30° Macula/and Affected Quadrant	60° 45° 30° *Sweep Periphery of Affected Quadrant (Document NVE) (Look for capillary non-perfusion)	60° 45° 30° *Macula/and Affected Quadrant (Document CME) (Document NVE)
POHS PRESUMED OCCULAR HISTOPLASMOSIS SYNDROME	30° Only *Macula/or Suspected Area of CNV (Clear FAZ important) (Look for early hyperfluorescence indicating CNV)	30° Macula/or Suspected Area of CNV	60° 45° 30° 20° Sweep Periphery (Document peripheral lesions — Histo Spots)	30° *Macula/or Suspected Area of CNV (Look for increased hyperfluorescence)
CSR CENTRAL SEROUS RETINOPATHY	30° Only *Macula (Clear FAZ important) (Look for 'Hot Spot' — pinpoint leak)	30° Macula	30° *Macula (Look for 'Smokestack' leak) Sweep Periphery	30° *Macula (Look for Increased Hyperfluorescence)
TUMOR	1° > Tumor *Affected Area (+ Disc if possible for orientation) (Stereo important)	1° > Tumor Affected Area (Stereo)	60° 45° 30° Affected Area (Stereo)	1° > Tumor *Affected Area (+ Disc if Possible) (Stereo)

Figure 7.7 Planning chart for properly sequencing angiograms. (Courtesy of Sheila Smith-Brewer, C.O.M.T., C.R.A.)

ticular disease. The beginner may need to use a medical dictionary to define some terms, but with some observation, explanation, and practice, the quality of work will improve along with an understanding of the typical pathologies most commonly photographed.

28. When switching eyes, shoot the macula first to alert the doctor that what follows is in the fellow eye. Include part of the optic disc in the photographs.

29. Begin to photograph the transit area at 7-10 seconds post-injection. The dye will first fill the choroid, then the arteries eminating from the optic disc. The dye then travels through arterioles, then capillaries, then venules to drain through the major veins exiting the optic disc. The major veins fill from edge to center (laminal flow). When the veins are completely filled move to the other eye and take a picture of the corresponding area of interest. Return to the principle transit eye and document other areas of interest (e.g., diabetic survey).
30. Take "late shots" at 10 minutes post-injection of the principle area of interest and the same area in the fellow eye.
31. Rewind and remove the film, then help the patient get up. Reassure the patient that all went well. Remind the patient about skin and urine discoloration, and send the patient back to the waiting area. Inform the doctor that you are finished. If your patient is an outside referral, give the patient some sunglasses and let the patient leave. If you are suspicious of a delayed reaction, allow the patient to sit in the waiting room for 20–30 minutes and doublecheck that all is well before sending the patient home.
32. Consult with the doctor about your initial observations whenever the patient may be "at risk", that is, if you suspect a subretinal neovascular membrane, or other pathology requiring immediate treatment.
33. Develop film ASAP when your index of suspicion is high.

The Photographer and the Doctor

The diagnostic role (area of responsibility) of the doctor is to order angiograms, to define the area of interest of the angiogram in chart notes and drawings or on a photo request form, examine and interpret the photographs and communicate the results to the patient.

The photographer's role is providing service to both the doctor and the patient; the doctor should, however, respect the photographer's experience. The photographer can often make the correct diagnosis. The photographer knows that doctors need immediate information for certain diagnoses and therefore should always notify the doctor as soon as possible when suspicious of threatening pathologies. The photographer must always be tactful when offering suggestions or warnings to the ophthalmologist, and speak as one professional to another. With the patient, the photographer must never usurp the doctor's role.

The photographer's communication with the ophthalmologist is every bit as important as communication with the patient.

When the patient presses for information, try any or all the following explanations:

- "The film sees more than the eye."
- "I have been concentrating on obtaining the best pictures I can."
- "This test is but one of several, and I would be doing you a disservice to guess at the diagnosis and/or prognosis based on one test."
- "It is the doctor's job to put together the pieces of the puzzle and to inform you. I am working on just one of the pieces."
- "I'll have to develop the film to get results."

As a general rule, speak politely to the patient, but refer all specific questions to the doctor about the results of the test.

At the same time, ask the doctor to review your work, explain what the doctor is looking for in each study, and why the information in the photographs is necessary or useful.

Angiography is a team effort. Keep the lines of communication open to optimize results for the patient.

What is needed to understand the proper sequencing of photographs is explained in the next section.

Dynamic Retinal Circulation in Fluorescein Angiography

Let X = the time dye travels from the patient's arm to eye. The phases or parts of an angiogram may be broken down as follows: (X usually equals 8-20 seconds).

1. Choroidal (X seconds postinjection). Dye arrival in the choroid and retina is a function of the blood circulation time in each patient, and will vary. In the prearterial phase you will see a choroidal background flush through the retinal pigment, as the choroidal vessels fill with dye (Figure 7.8).
2. Retinal arterial filling is next (X + 1–2 seconds). The arteries fill centrally first, then peripherally radiating out from the optic disc. This event often occurs too fast to record unless you begin taking pictures before the dye arrives in the eye (Figure 7.8).
3. Next is capillary filling or the filling of the very small arteries and veins, both around the fovea and in the peripheral capillaries (X + 3 seconds). These small vessels are not normally visible with white light; they are best seen in the capillary net around the foveal

The five phases of an angiogram are the choroidal, arterial, capillary, venous, and late phase. A good angiogram contains all five phases, as well as early and late photographs of the fellow eye. Begin photography before the dye reaches the eye to ensure capturing the choroidal and arterial phases.

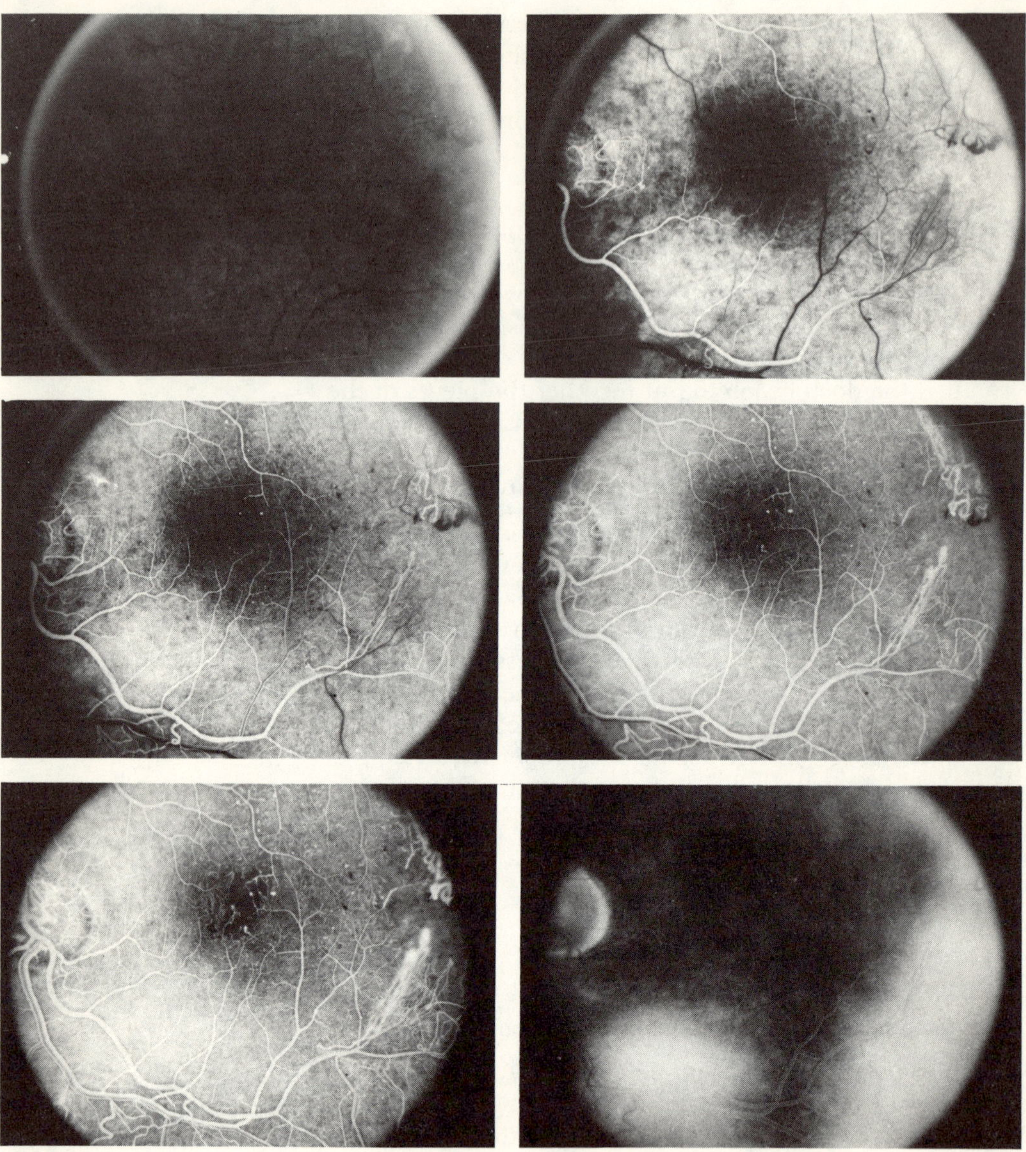

Figure 7.8 The six phases of an angiogram (patient is diabetic): Choroidal (top left). Arterial (top right). Early capillary (center left). Early venous (center right). Mid venous (bottom left). Late (bottom right). Filling stages often overlap due to the pathology involved or variations in filling patterns.

avascular zone. Both centrally and peripherally these capillaries fill and begin to return the dye through the venules to the veins (Figure 7.8).

4. Next is the early venous phase (X + 5 seconds) in which the veins fill at the edges first, then gradually fill to the center. This laminal filling occurs in arteries and veins. Arterial filling is so rapid that it is hard to photograph. Venous filling is slower and easier to record. Laminal flow occurs because the flow speed of blood at the center of a vein is faster than at its edges (Figure 7.8).
5. Next is full venous phase (X + 10 seconds) in which laminar filling is completed. Constant pumping of the

heart will make the arteries, then the veins, briefly shine brightly again as the dye recirculates dye stained blood continuously through arteries and veins in the retina. Often this "recirculation phase" is difficult to see in the camera or on film (Figure 7.8).

6. The final phase is the late phase (X + 10–15 minutes). These are photos taken 10 minutes postinjection. These photos are used for comparison with early transit photos to differentiate different dye patterns in the eye. In a normal angiogram dye has mixed with blood to a point where it almost ceases to be observable by the photographer (Figure 7.8).

Seeing these phases in the camera eyepiece is secondary to recording them on the film. While interpretation of angiograms is outside the scope of this book, a vocabulary of interpretation of normal and abnormal fundus fluorescence is useful to the photographer (especially those seeking to become Certified Retinal Angiographers [C.R.A.]) Ask your ophthalmologist for books to read on this subject if it interests you.

Types of Fluorescence—Normal and Abnormal

The following section on fluorescence is more a roadmap to determine where you are and where you are going when you perform fluorescein angiography, than a guide to interpretation.

The interpretation of angiograms is the doctor's job. Taking the correct pictures for the doctor to interpret, however, is the photographer's job. The photographer must know what is normal and what is not when performing an angiogram.

Normal fluorescence means dye doing what it should do. Abnormal fluorescence is simply a dye pattern breaking the normal rules.

There are two vascular supplies in the fundus. One is the choroidal blood supply. The choroid's blood vessels normally leak fluorescein dye. The blood vessel walls have fenestration, or windows, which allow fluorescein to leak out and stain the serous fluid surrounding the choroidal vessels. In a normal angiogram the choroidal vessels fill first, and gradually leak dye until in late phase they empty of dye, turning dark again in a sea of fluorescein stained serous fluid.

The second vascular system is the retinal blood vessels of the neurosensory retina, the eye's film. These blood vessels *normally* do not leak dye. Their vessel walls contain tight cell junctions through which fluorescein molecules cannot pass. These blood vessels fill seconds after the choroidal vessels fill. In a normal angiogram the retinal vessels fill then empty of dye. The retinal pigment epithelium (RPE) is a barrier to fluorescence between these two vascular systems. The higher the melanin pigment in RPE cells the greater the barrier effect. In the lightly pigmented eye normal choroidal fluorescence is easy to observe.

The optic nerve head has a capillary circulation connected to the choroidal circulation. The optic disc capillaries normally leak dye. In the late phase of the angiogram, the optic disk may have a halo of fluorescence surrounding its edges, or even stain completely in the normal eye. Look for this landmark when taking late phase photographs.

The normal fluorescein patterns and vascular dynamics just presented are the normal standard against which variations in fluorescence are weighed to interpret the abnormal angiogram. Interpretation is simply knowing what is normal in angiographic studies and what is not, and describing the difference.

Certain types of fluorescence patterns repeat themselves over and over in fluorescein angiograms. Acquiring the vocabulary of these patterns will improve the quality of studies the photographer performs.

Normal fluorescence is maintained only by continuous excitation of the dye by the flashes of blue light from the camera. Each camera flash excites the dye briefly as serial photographs are taken. In the absence of dye, no fluorescence should be recorded, but as seen earlier, both autofluorescence and pseudofluorescence can occur in photos taken prior to a dye injection (Figure 7.3). These conditions must be taken into account when interpreting angiograms. Often such information is only available on the original negatives.

The four principle types of abnormal hyperfluorescence are
1) staining
2) leakage
3) pooling
4) transmission

If there is too much fluorescence it is called hyperfluorescence. Hyperfluorescence can be normal, as when the sclera stains from the dye in the choroidal serous fluid, or abnormal in four different ways. The four types of abnormal hyperfluorescence are: staining, leakage, pooling, and transmission. In almost every case these mechanisms occur in combination or in sequence rather than as unique separate patterns. The leakage of dye from an abnormal blood vessel will stain tumor tissue and pool in the fluid surrounding the tumor. Figure 7.9 demonstrates classic examples of conditions in which each one of the four types of hyperfluorescence is dominant.

Staining of tissue by fluorescein dye is comparable to staining a rug with red wine. The tumor tissue absorbs dye molecules and fluoresces in the later phases of the angiogram (Figure 7.9). Leakage and pooling are also occuring.

Leakage occurs either from inside a blood vessel to outside the vessel wall or from one anatomic layer of the fundus to another, ie choroid to neurosensory retina.

Vascular leakage is demonstrated in a diabetic patient with new blood vessel growth, that is, retinal neovascularization (Figure 7.9). These new blood vessels in the retina, like

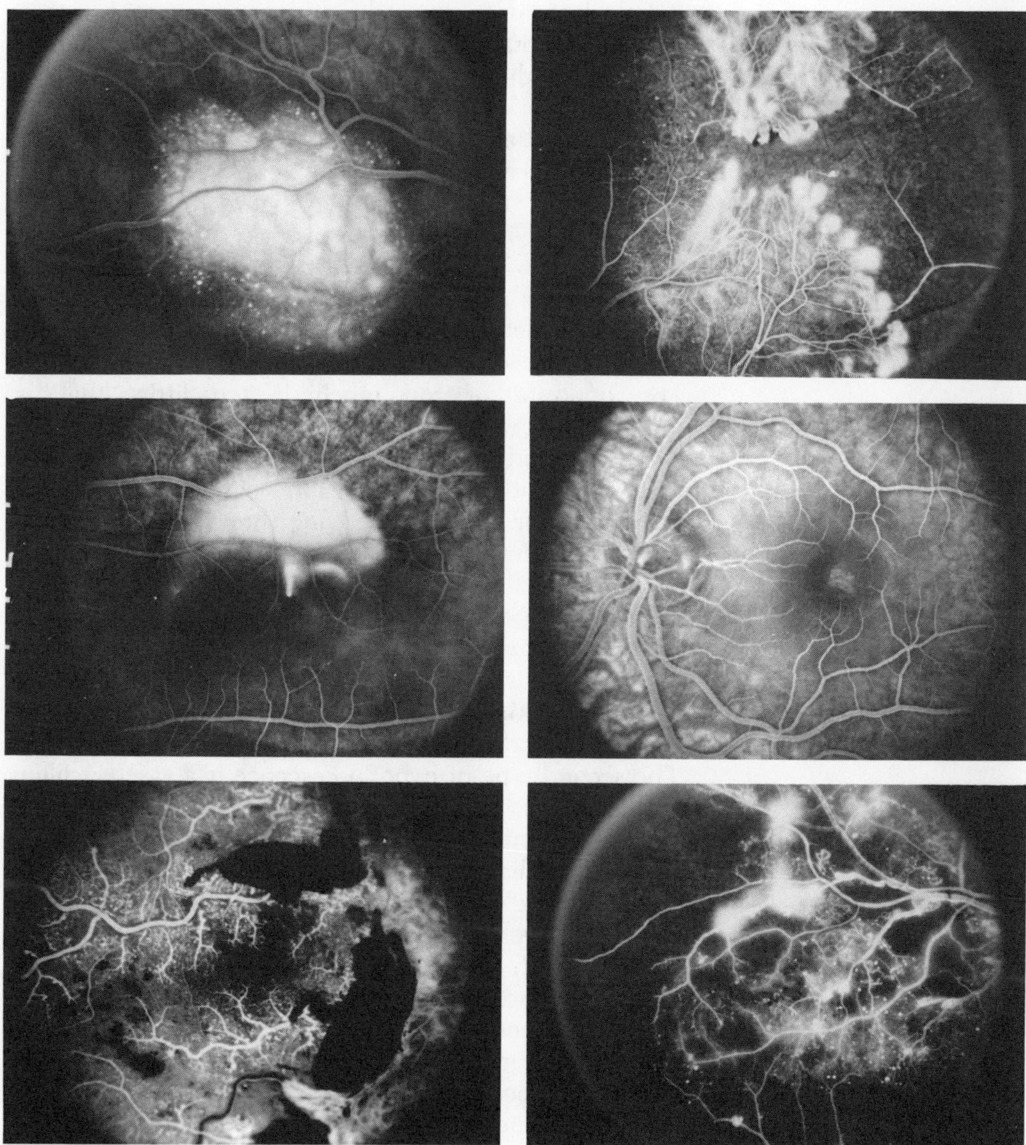

Figure 7.9 The four hyperfluorescence patterns: Staining—of an ocular tumor (top left). Leakage—from diabetic neovascularization (top right). Pooling—of dye in a patient with central serous choroidopathy (center left). Transmission—of dye in a fovea with pigmentary disruption (center right). The two hypofluorescence patterns: Blockage due to intraretinal blood (bottom left). Nonperfusion of dye in areas of absent retinal capillaries (bottom right).

choroidal vessels, leak dye through their walls. Another form of neovascularization demonstrating leakage from one anatomic layer to another is the growth of small choroidal vessels through the RPE and under the sensory retina. This subretinal neovascular blood vessel leaks dye and serous fluid into a confined blister-like area, and pooling of leaked dye will occur late in the angiogram.

Pooling of dye occurs in any retinal area of defined dimensions in which a normally leaking blood vessel or serous fluid is present. The choroid normally pools dye. Any break in retinal pigment cells can allow serous fluid to pass through the RPE into the subsensory retinal space. This condition is called central serous choroidopathy, (Figure 7.9). With an active "hole in the dike," the leaking dye in the choroidal serous fluid passes through the RPE into the blister under the sensory retina gradually filling the blister with dye, that is, pooling.

Any area of absent RPE will allow normal choroidal fluorescence to be transmitted through this "window defect" and be seen by the photographer (Figure 7.9). Early in the angiogram this window will appear bright, but as dye intensity diminishes with time, this brightness will fade. Late photographs are always necessary to differentiate between an increase or decrease in an area of abnormal fluorescence as a study proceeds.

The opposite of too much is too little, that is, hypofluorescence. Normal hypofluorescence occurs in the darkly pigmented areas of the fundus. The foveal RPE cells are thicker, with greater melanin concentration. Such pigmentation blocks the underlying choroidal fluorescence. A darkly pigmented fundus blocks choroidal fluorescence throughout the fundus.

Abnormal hypofluorescencies of two types. The first is blockage. Blood is a barrier to fluorescence. Any areas of blood will block the underlying fluorescence (Figure 7.9). Certain nonvascular fibrous tissue growths can also mask fluorescence, as does melanin in the RPE.

The second type of hypofluorescence is a vascular filling defect. Such filling defects are produced by either delays or the absence of perfusion of the retinal or choroidal vasculature. In the diabetic patient, for example, ischemia, the closure of blood vessels (usually capillaries) occurs. These areas of dead vessels demonstrate no vasculature where it should be. Such areas fail to perfuse with dye. These are areas of hypofluorescence.

The two principle types of abnormal hypofluorescence are 1) blockage and 2) nonperfusion—nonfilling or delayed filling of intra or extra vascular spaces.

Recognize these six abnormal patterns. They occur in combination in many pathological conditions. Hypofluorescent areas can be immediately adjacent to hyperfluorescent areas in the same eye. Whenever in doubt, take a picture. Film is much cheaper than an ignored area of pathology.

Summary

Remember, the angiogram is an ancillary diagnostic test. The doctor initially evaluates a patient's retina, determines the need for more information, and orders a fluorescein angiogram. The analysis of intra and extravascular fluorescence, however, can be a significant tool for the best possible diagnosis, treatment, and prognosis for the patient.

A consistent form of analysis or interpretation is as essential to derive as much information as necessary from each angiogram as are the images produced to make these interpretations. The photographer's job is to maximize the information of the film for the doctor's use and the patient's benefit.

Many good books have been written about fluorescein angiography interpretation. These books analyze pictures of the specific diseases you as a photographer will be asked to document with your fundus camera.

Review these books to learn more about your photographic subject, and further understand descriptive interpretation.

Two good starting points are books by

Gass, Donald. Stereoscopic Atlas of Macular Disease. CW Mosby, 1988.

Schatz, Howard. Essentials of Fluorescein Angiography. Pacific Press, 1983.

Ask your physician for other texts she or he may have in her/his library.

CHAPTER 8

Black-and-White Film Processing

by J. Michael Coppinger

While not all retinal or ophthalmic photographers process their own films, knowing how to process the black-and-white films is both useful, and sometimes, necessary. This brief chapter explains film processing, then outlines the procedure for processing black-and-white film.

Developing Black-and-White Film

The development process is the chemical means of making the invisible image stored on the exposed film a visible permanent image. Four basic steps occur in this process:

- Development, in which the silver nitrates in the film are converted back to metallic silver. This process is then stopped with water or glacial acetic acid.
- Fixation, in which the nonexposed, still light sensitive silver is removed from the film. Once fixation is complete, the film may be exposed to light.
- Washing, to remove the residual fixer from the film.
- Drying the film.

Black-and-white negative development can be easily done in the office. Take a trip to a local professional photography store with a list of supplies you will need. Talk to a salesperson and examine the equipment you want before purchasing it.

Film development is always done for a fixed time at a specific temperature. Time and temperature are inversely related. As temperature decreases, time of development increases (or vice versa). Monitoring film development temperature is critical for consistent results. All chemicals should be used at the same temperature. Sudden shifts in temperature from one chemical to the next can damage the film.

To process black-and-white film you will need the following supplies: a film developing tank, scissors, a light-tight room or a changing bag (a double-lined light-tight bag into which you place both arms to load the film), reels to hold the film in the developing tank (Figure 8.1), a thermometer, a sink with running water, the chemicals necessary to develop

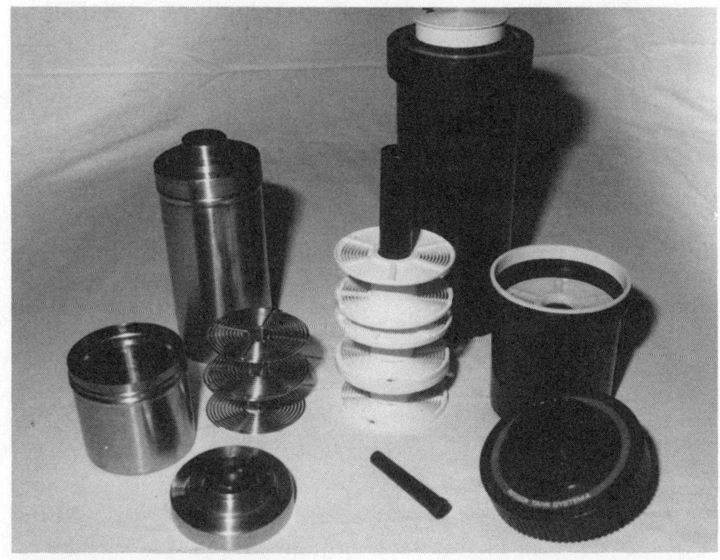

Figure 8.1 A steel reel film developing system on the 'eft, a plastic reel system on the right.

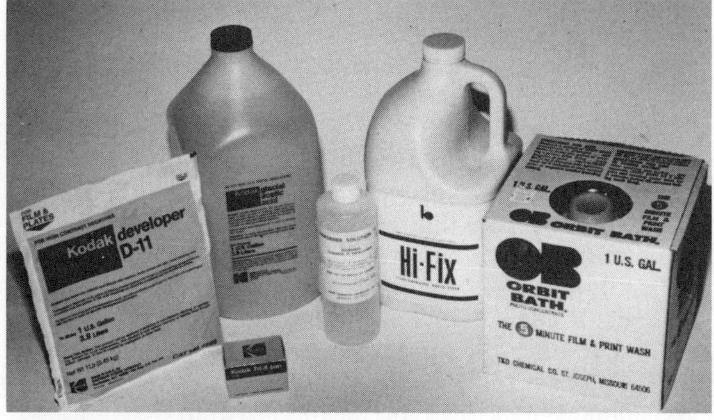

Figure 8.2 A complete set of chemicals for black-and-white film processing—(left to right) HC-110 liquid developer, D-19 powder developer, Glacial acetic acid stop bath, Kodak Rapid Fixer, Hypocheck, Permawash and photo-flo.

the film (Figure 8.2), and a clock to time each development stage.

When loading film on reels in a changing bag, the developing tank must be in the changing bag. Load the reels. Place the reels in the developing tank and secure its lid. After removing from the changing bag, pour the developer into the tank through the hole in the lid. (Bang the tank on the counter to remove trapped air bubbles.)

Step-by-Step Film Processing

In a light-tight room with the lights on:

1. Set the film cassettes, scissors, can opener, film reels and developing tank's center post on a dry table.
2. Set the developing tank and the developer in the sink. Pour developer into the tank and measure the

Film developing tank and reels are available in steel and plastic types. Film reel loading is easier with the plastic system than with the steel, but plastic developing tanks are fragile and can break. Try both systems with a blank roll of film at a photography store before selecting a system for use.

temperature. Calculate the development time and set the timer appropriately.

3. Turn off the room lights. Wait a few minutes to dark adapt to see if there are any light leaks around door or windows. Cover these leaks before opening film cassettes.
4. Load the film onto the reels.
5. Place the film into the tank and agitate it for 30 seconds.
6. Cover the developing tank with the lid (securely) and turn the lights on.
7. Agitate the tank regularly for 15 seconds each minute during the time required for development. Some film manufacturers recommend agitating for 5 seconds each 30 seconds. Consistency is what counts.
8. Pour the developer back into its bottle or discard it at the end of the development period. Later mark the new number of rolls processed on the cap if reusing the developer.
9. Stop development. The tank lid remains on. Rinse off the film in the developing tank for one minute with running water. Fill the tank with water, then pour it out again. Do this 4–6 times. An alternative is to use glacial acetic acid as a stop bath. Pour the stop bath into the tank, then agitate for 30 seconds. Pour the stop bath back into its bottle through a funnel.
10. Fix the film. The tank lid is still on the developing tank. Pour the film fixer into the developing tank. The fixer removes the unexposed silver from the film. Agitate the tank for the first thirty seconds, then fix it for 2–5 more minutes, agitating fifteen seconds per minute. Different fixers require different times. Check the fixer you are using for time recommendations. When fixation is complete, check the fixer for exhaustion with a hypocheck solution, then pour the fixer from the developing tank back into the fixer bottle if it is still good. If the fixer is exhausted, discard it, and refix the film with fresh fixer.

    Now it is ok to take the lid off the developing tank.
11. Rinse the film again in the developing tank with running water for at least 1 minute, filling then dumping the tank.
12. Pour a hypoeliminator into the tank and agitate the film constantly for two minutes. This chemical eliminates the fixer and reduces washing time.

13. Pour the hypoeliminator back into its bottle, and wash the film for 3–5 minutes, again, filling and dumping continuously.
14. Add a ½ capful of Photo-flo solution to the tank filled with water. Agitate the film for 30 seconds. This solution reduces the surface tension of the water on the film, and prevents spotting while the film dries.
15. Remove the film from the reels and hang the film to dry in a dust free area. Film drying cabinets with heater fans speed this process, but are relatively expensive for in-office processing.
16. When the film is dry, cut the negatives into strips and store them in plastic sleeves. Mark the patient's name on the film sleeve.

Film Development Recommendations

Many different chemical developers are used for processing black and white film. One universal developer, good for fluorescein angiograms and specular microscopy done on 400 ASA black and white film, is Kodak's D-11 Developer.

An alternative, Kodak HC-110 Developer comes in liquid rather than powder form, and is easier to mix for developing.

The following table is only a guide, as each camera system needs different amounts of light to expose the negatives properly and therefore may require different development times.

Fluorescein Tri-X Film Processing in D-11

(Using a Zeiss FF-3 fundus camera, flash setting for exposure equal to 150 watt/seconds.)

Development Time	Chemical Temperature
nine minutes	65°
eight minutes	68°
seven minutes	70°
six minutes	72°

This development chart lists times and temperatures for one particular developer, Kodak D–11. Other developers will process angiograms effectively. The other most commonly used developer is HC–110. Use Dilution A, which is explained on the developer bottle. Development times and temperatures are similar to those for D–11. Run a test roll before processing a batch of angiograms.

To reuse the developer, mark the top of the D-11 bottle with the number of rolls already processed. *Add* the following time to each batch, based on the number of rolls already processed to compensate for chemical energy lost by the developer with successive uses.

At 65°, 10.8 seconds X roll already processed.
At 68°, 9.6 seconds X roll already processed.
At 70°, 8.4 seconds X roll already processed.
At 72°, 7.2 seconds X roll already processed.

(Example: 15 rolls already processed, the developing temperature is 68°. Multiply 15 x 9.6 = 144 seconds or 2 minutes 24 seconds. Add 2 minutes 24 seconds to the initial developing time of 8 minutes. The total time for developing is 10 minutes and 24 seconds.)

Discard the developer when you reach 35 + rolls processed, as this is the capacity of D–11. *Always* filter the used developer through cotton when pouring it back into the D–11 bottle. This eliminates the sludge produced by the developer's chemical action on the film, and extends developer life.

Use plastic bottles. Squeeze the air out of the plastic bottles to prolong the life of the developer, because oxygen in the bottle will reduce the potency of the developer. Discard half full bottles of developer unused for more than one month and mix fresh developer. Mark the date the developer is mixed on the bottle.

Diluting Developers

HC-110 developer is diluted for use, then discarded. Use Dilution A as directed on the bottle—1 part working solution to three parts water.

Developer can be mixed 1:1 with water in a dilute solution. Development time must be doubled and the developer discarded after one use. All other steps in the development process are as outlined. Dilution is a good way to control temperature. Do not dilute other chemicals other than directed on the container.

Summary

In this brief chapter, black-and-white film processing is outlined. The subsequent process of making positive contact prints or photographic enlargements is described in many general photography texts. Read such a book for more information.

Specular and angiographic negatives are easily interpreted in original negative form by ophthalmologists. In-office processing allows speedy interpretation and improved patient care. Black-and-white print development follows the same chemical process as film development. If the doctor can be convinced to read negatives much time is saved by the photographer, and much money by the doctor, as only a common sink is necessary to develop film.

Additional Sources of Information

The authors have elected to provide the reader with a brief list of comprehensive texts currently available rather than an extensive and generally inaccessible list of bibliographical material. These books cover ophthalmic anatomy, physiology, general photography, scientific photography, and specialized areas of ophthalmic photography. Many other sources can be found in medical libraries and through photographic book dealers. One overlooked source is the ophthalmologist's library in your own office.

Blaker, Alfred, R.P.B. *Handbook for Scientific Photography.* San Francisco: W.H. Freeman and Company, 1977.

Davson, H. *Physiology of the Eye.* 4th ed. Orlando: Academic Press, 1980.

Dorland's Illustrated Medical Dictionary. 26th ed. Philadelphia: W.B. Saunders Company, 1985.

Duane, Thomas D., M.D., Ph.D., Ed., and Edward A. Jaeger, M.D., Asst. Ed. *Clinical Ophthalmology.* Philadelphia: Harper & Row Publishers, 1982.

Hedgecoe, John. *The Book of Photography.* New York: Alfred A. Knopf, 1984.

Justice, Johnny, Jr., C.R.A., F.O.P.S. *Ophthalmic Photography.* Boston: Little, Brown & Co., 1982.

Martonyi, Csaba, C.R.A., F.O.P.S., Charles Bahn, M.D., and Robert Meyer, M.D. *Clinical Slit Lamp Biomicroscopy and Photo Slit Lamp Biomicrography.* Ann Arbor: Time One Ink Ltd.

Mayer, Daniel, M.D. *Clinical Wide Field Specular Microscopy.* London: Tindall, Bailliere, 1984.

Vaughan, Daniel, Taylor Asbury, and Robert Cook. *General Ophthalmology.* 10th ed. Los Altos, California: Lange Medical Publications, 1983.

Wong, Don, R.B.P., F.O.P.S. *Textbook of Ophthalmic Photography.* Ambler, Pennsylvania: InterOptics Publishers, 1982.

Index

Fixation, 14
Flash photography, 28
Flash synchronization, 8